Mahmood Ahmad

Sustained release formulation development by microencapsulation

Ghulam Murtaza
Mahmood Ahmad

Sustained release formulation development by microencapsulation

Formulation development, characterization and in vitro-in vivo correlation development

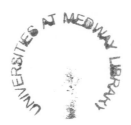

LAP LAMBERT Academic Publishing

Impressum/Imprint (nur für Deutschland/ only for Germany)

Bibliografische Information der Deutschen Nationalbibliothek: Die Deutsche Nationalbibliothek verzeichnet diese Publikation in der Deutschen Nationalbibliografie; detaillierte bibliografische Daten sind im Internet über http://dnb.d-nb.de abrufbar.

Alle in diesem Buch genannten Marken und Produktnamen unterliegen warenzeichen-, marken- oder patentrechtlichem Schutz bzw. sind Warenzeichen oder eingetragene Warenzeichen der jeweiligen Inhaber. Die Wiedergabe von Marken, Produktnamen, Gebrauchsnamen, Handelsnamen, Warenbezeichnungen u.s.w. in diesem Werk berechtigt auch ohne besondere Kennzeichnung nicht zu der Annahme, dass solche Namen im Sinne der Warenzeichen- und Markenschutzgesetzgebung als frei zu betrachten wären und daher von jedermann benutzt werden dürften.

Coverbild: www.ingimage.com

Verlag: LAP LAMBERT Academic Publishing GmbH & Co. KG
Dudweiler Landstr. 99, 66123 Saarbrücken, Deutschland
Telefon +49 681 3720-310, Telefax +49 681 3720-3109
Email: info@lap-publishing.com

Herstellung in Deutschland:
Schaltungsdienst Lange o.H.G., Berlin
Books on Demand GmbH, Norderstedt
Reha GmbH, Saarbrücken
Amazon Distribution GmbH, Leipzig
ISBN: 978-3-8383-8412-2

Imprint (only for USA, GB)

Bibliographic information published by the Deutsche Nationalbibliothek: The Deutsche Nationalbibliothek lists this publication in the Deutsche Nationalbibliografie; detailed bibliographic data are available in the Internet at http://dnb.d-nb.de.

Any brand names and product names mentioned in this book are subject to trademark, brand or patent protection and are trademarks or registered trademarks of their respective holders. The use of brand names, product names, common names, trade names, product descriptions etc. even without a particular marking in this works is in no way to be construed to mean that such names may be regarded as unrestricted in respect of trademark and brand protection legislation and could thus be used by anyone.

Cover image: www.ingimage.com

Publisher: LAP LAMBERT Academic Publishing GmbH & Co. KG
Dudweiler Landstr. 99, 66123 Saarbrücken, Germany
Phone +49 681 3720-310, Fax +49 681 3720-3109
Email: info@lap-publishing.com

Printed in the U.S.A.
Printed in the U.K. by (see last page)
ISBN: 978-3-8383-8412-2

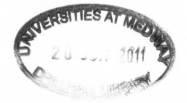

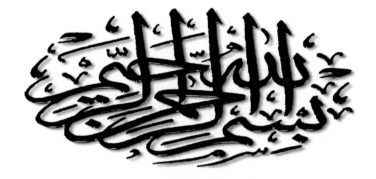

In the Name of Allah, the Most Merciful, the Most Kind.

Dedication

To

My Mother, Father, Uncle (Rashid Ahmad) & Research Supervisor

Who Always Pray, Love, Support and Encourage Me

Certificate

It is hereby certified that work presented by Ghulam Murtaza S/O Habib Ahmad in the dissertation entitled "formulation development of salbutamol by microencapsulation, its in-vitro and in-vivo studies" has been successfully carried out under my supervision in partial fulfillment of the requirements for the degree of Doctor of philosophy (Pharmaceutics) in the Department of Pharmacy, Faculty of Pharmacy and Alternative Medicines, The Islamia University of Bahawalpur.

Prof. Dr. Mahmood Ahmad
Supervisor,
Faculty of Pharmacy and Alternative Medicines,
The Islamia University of Bahawalpur.

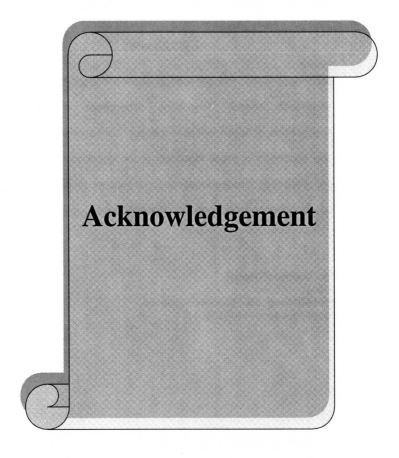

Acknowledgement

Acknowledgement

I have no words to express my deepest gratitude to Almighty, Compassionate, and Supreme **Allah**, who enable me to accomplish this task. I also invoke peace for **Hazrat Muhammad (SAW)**, the Last Prophet of Allah, who is forever a torch of guidance for humanity as a whole.

I express my gratitude to all my teachers whose teachings have brought me to this stage of academic zenith but in particular I wish to express immeasurable gratitude to my supervisor **Prof. Dr. Mahmood Ahmad**, Dean, Faculty of Pharmacy and Alternative Medicine, the Islamia University of Bahawalpur, for his quick brave decisions and very kind attitude. It was a wonderful experience to work under his supervision. His intellect guided me to overcome all barriers in research. His indefatigable patience made me believe that everything is easy. His kind supervision and help enabled me to complete this report rather a difficult task.

Without cooperation of **Dr. Nisar-ur-Rehman**, Chairman, Department of Pharmacy & Dr. Naveed Akhtar, Associate Professor, Department of Pharmacy, it was impossible for me to fulfill my objective as they introduced me to the good senses of research.

I can't forget efforts of all my submissive research fellows, Muhammad Waheed Asghar, Muhammad Asadullah Madni, Usman Menhas, Muhammad Akhtar Raees, Muhammad Rizwan, Fahad Perwaiz, Muhammad Atif, Shujaat Ali Khan, Muhammad Naeem Aamir, Shoaib Ali Khan, Mrs. Fatima Shoaib, Muhammad Yaqoob Saqi, Muhammad Sarfraz Khalil, Zubair Malik, Wajid Hussain, Shaiq-uz-Zaman and Ramzi Hussain Shawahna for my research and thesis.

Many warmest thanks for Dr. Raimar Loebenberg, Associate Professor, Faculty of Pharmacy, University of Alberta for encouraging me when ever I was in tension and for giving me something else to think about.

In the last but not the least, I pay my deepest respect to my family especially my elder brother, Ghulam Mustafa and my wife, Munazza Ejaz whose love and affection kept me steadfast and enabled me to attain targets and goal of academic life. They always encouraged me at each level. I express my deepest gratitude to the cute and attractive smile of my dear innocent daughter, Urwa Murtaza, which always refreshes me when ever I am very tired during this exhausting effort.

Ghulam Murtaza

Manuscripts Accepted for Publications in HEC
Approved / Impact Factor Journals

1. Murtaza G., Ahmad M., Madni M. A., Asghar M. W. Optimization and validation of a new and sensitive reverse phase hplc method with fluorescent detection for the determination of salbutamol sulfate in human plasma. Bull. Chem. Soc. Ethop. April 2009, 23(01), 001-008 (In Press).

2. Murtaza G., Ahmad M. Microencapsulation of Tramadol hydrochloride and Physicochemical Evaluation of Formulations. Accepted for publication in Pak. J. Chem. Soc. June 2009 (In Press).

3. Ghulam Murtaza, Mahmood Ahmad, Muhammad Waheed Asghar and Muhammad Naeem Aamir. Salbutamol sulphate-ethylcellulose microparticles: formulation and in-vitro evaluation with emphasis on mathematical approaches. Accepted for publication in DARU. June 2009 (In Press).

4. Ghulam Murtaza, Mahmood Ahmad, Naveed Akhtar, Fatima Rasool. A comparative study of various microencapsulation techniques: effect of polymer viscosity on microcapsule characteristics. Accepted for publication in Pak. J. Pharm. Sci. 2009 (In Press).

5. Ghulam Murtaza, Murtaza Ahmad, Gul Shehnaz. Microencapsulation of diclofenac sodium by non-solvent addition technique: Use of toluene and petroleum benzin as solvent and non-solvent respectively. Accepted for publication in Tropical Journal of Pharmaceutical Research.

List of Abbreviations

Abbreviations	Meaning
SS	Salbutamol Sulphate
TH	Tramadol Hydrochloride
DS	Diclofenac Sodium
EC	Ethylcellulose
SE	Solvent Evaporation
CNSA	Coacervation Non-solvent Addition
CTC	Coacervation Thermal Change
BP	British Pharmacopoeia
USP	United States Pharmacopoeia
M	Microparticles
T	Tablets
TA	Thermal Analysis
XRD	X-Ray Diffractometry
FTIR	Fourier Transform Infra-red
UV	Ultraviolet
SEM	Scanning Electron Microscope
DSC	Differential Scanning Calorimetry
TGA	Thermogravimetric Analysis
DTA	Differential Thermal Analysis
HPLC	High Performance Liquid Chromatography
IVIVC	In vitro – In vivo Correlation
C_{max}	Maximum Plasma Concentration
T_{max}	Time to Reach Maximum Plasma Concentration
AUC	Area Under Curve
SD	Standard Deviation
cp	Centipoise
BCS	Biopharmaceutical classification System
HPMC	Hydroxypropylmethylcellulose
PIB	Polyisobutylene

LIST OF CONTENTS

LIST OF TABLES

LIST OF FIGURES

LIST OF REPORTS

AIMS AND OBJECTIVES

1. To microencapsulate salbutamol sulpahte into the ethylcellulose coats using non-solvent addition coacervation technique.

2. To apply non-solvent addition coacervation technique for the microencapsulation of drugs with different solubilities (Tramadol hydrochloride, salbutamol sulphate and diclofenac sodium) into ethylcellulose coats and compare the formulations.

3. To find the sources of variation in entrapment efficiency, production yield, mean particle size and the drug release behavior among the formulations.

4. To investigate any possible chemical interaction between drugs and polymer.

5. To test the potential application of ethylcellulose microparticles as a suitable sustained release drug delivery system.

6. To compare physical properties of microcapsules prepared by three techniques i.e. coacervation-non solvent addition, coacervation-thermal change and solvent evaporation.

7. To develop, optimize and validate a new sensitive and specific reverse phase-high performance liquid chromatography method for salbutamol sulphate estimation in human plasma using fluorescent detector and isocratic elution.

8. To investigate biowaiver study of tabletted microparticles of salbutamol sulphate (a BCS class I drug).

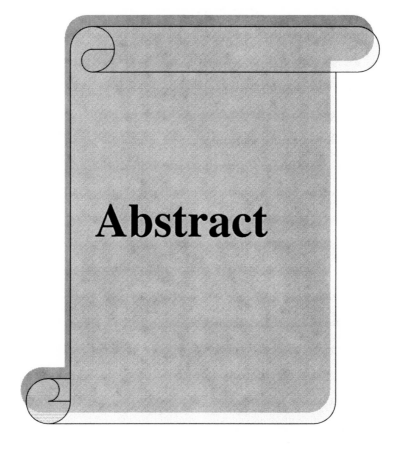

Abstract

ABSTRACT

This report provides chemistry of salbutamol sulphate, tramadol hydrochloride, diclofenac sodium and ethylcellulose, physics of drug release through particle wall and use of microparticles in life sciences. Microparticles of salbutamol sulphate were prepared by using three different microencapsulation techniques i.e. coacervation thermal change, solvent evaporation and coacervation non-solvent addition by adjusting the ratio of drug to ethylcellulose. Salbutamol sulphate microparticles were compared with the microparticles of diclofenac sodium and tramadol hydrochloride and characterized by micromeritics, SEM, FTIR, X-RD, dissolution and thermal studies. The microcapsules were then compressed into tablets to study the variation of drug release between microcapsules and tabletted microcapsules. In vitro release profiles of prepared microcapsules and tabletted microcapsules were studied using USP XXIV dissolution apparatus I and II, respectively, in 450 ml double distilled water at 50 rpm maintained at 37°C. Microparticles were whitish, irregular in morphology and aggregated with good stability, fine rheological properties and excellent encapsulation efficiency. Percentage yield was almost greater than 90% in each batch. Initial burst effect was observed in the release pattern of tramadol hydrochloride and salbutamol sulphate formulations. No strong chemical interaction was observed between the drugs and polymer in microparticles. The release of drug from their respective formulations was sustained in the following rank: diclofenac sodium > salbutamol sulphate > tramadol hydrochloride. Polymer concentration and sustained release behavior were found to be directly proportional to each other. A slight increase in actual drug loading but profound increase in mean diameter of microcapsules was observed with an increase in the viscosity of ethylcellulose. The rate of drug release from microparticles decreased as the concentration of polyisobutylene was increased from 6% to 12% during microencapsulation. UV and FTIR spectroscopy, x-ray diffractometry and thermal analysis showed that ethylcellulose did not interact with these drugs. The release pattern of tabletted microparticles was affected significantly ($p < 0.05$) by the addition of HPMC as excepient and insignificantly ($p > 0.05$) by the type of dissolution media and stirring speed. All the batches of tablets showed good stability and reproducibility. Release profiles were evaluated by model-dependent and model independent approaches. The drug release from all the formulations was best explained by Higuchi's equation, as the plots showed highest linearity, followed by zero order and first order. The mechanism of drug release was anomalous diffusion from all formulations. Non-solvent addition phase separation was found to be a suitable method to develop ethylcellulose based multi-unit controlled release drug delivery system.

A sensitive reverse phase-high performance liquid chromatography (RP-HPLC) method with fluorescent detector (FLD) was developed and optimized for salbutamol sulfate determination in human plasma. In this regard, mobile phase specifications, extraction procedures, excitation and emission wavelengths were optimized. The HPLC system consisted of a Lichrosorb RP-C18 analytical column (4.6 × 200 mm, 5 µm) with FLD operated at excitation 228 nm and emission 310 nm. Mobile phase {CH_3OH / $(NH_4)H_2PO_4$ (67 mM)(pH 3.0) / Triethylamine (TEA), 50 / 50 / 0.02 (v/v/v%)} was run at a flow rate of 0.7 mL/min. To clean up samples, a liquid-liquid extraction (LLE) procedure was selected and optimized. Salbutamol sulphate and tramadol hydrochloride eluted at 4.1 and 5.2 minutes respectively. Adequate extraction efficiency was achieved by DEHP (75.88-85.52%). The standard curve was linear for the range tested (0.5–80 ng/mL) and the coefficient of determination was 0.9989. A detection limit of 0.17 ng/mL was achieved. The intra- and inter-day precision was less than 4%. The present assay combines adequate accuracy and precision with sensitivity for salbutamol sulphate determination in human plasma and can be applied to study pharmacokinetics of salbutamol sulphate sustained release tablets after oral administration in human.

A good linear correlation (R^2 = 0.9224, 0.945, 0.9363 and 0.9694 for T_1, T_2, T_3 and reference formulations, respectively) was obtained between the percent cumulative drug released (in vitro) and the percent cumulative drug absorbed (in vivo) data of these formulations at specific time points to develop level A in vitro-in vivo correlation that shows a reliable prediction of the plasma concentrations obtained following a single dose.

Keywords:

Coacervation, Solvent evaporation, Viscosity grade, Salbutamol sulphate, Tramadol hydrochloride, Dissolution, Diclofenac sodium, Ethylcellulose, Characterization, Method optimization, RP-HPLC method, Fluorescent detection, Ion-pair extraction, Calibration curve, Internal standard, In-vitro and in-vivo correlation.

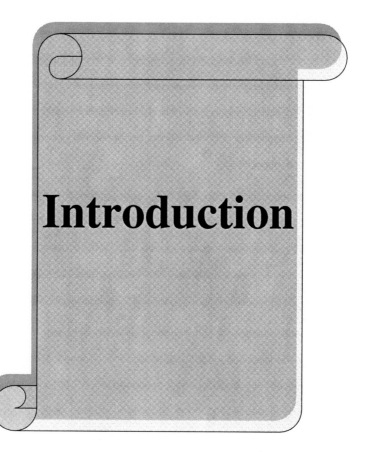

Introduction

1. INTRODUCTION

The number of patients with chronic diseases is increasing day by day. This situation necessitates the development of drugs for a longer period and taking a lot of medicines simultaneously, which can lead to a decrease in patient compliance. This problem is serious for drugs with short biological half lives because they must be taken more frequently. One method to solve such problems is to develop a dosage form capable of releasing the drug gradually. In this regard, microencapsulation has been used as one of the methods to construct a formulation for delivering the drug in a controlled mode (Yamuda et al. 2001). Microencapsulation is the application of a thin coating to individual core materials that have an arbitrary particle size range from 5-5000 μm (Bakan 1986).

Salbutamol sulphate (SS, Bis[(1RS)-2-[(1,1-dimethylethyl)amino]-1-[4-hydroxy-3-(hydroxymethyl)phenyl] ethanol] sulphate, $[(C_{13}H_{21}NO_3)_2.H_2So_4]$, Figure-1.1) is a potent β_2-adrenoceptor stimulant which is used for the treatment of reversible airways obstruction. It is readily absorbed from the gastrointestinal tract when administered orally. Its biological half life is about 4 to 6 hours (Martindale 2002).

Tramadol hydrochloride (TH, Figure-1.2) is a centrally acting analgesic having both opioid and non-opioid effects (Lee et al., 1993). It is indicated when non steroidal anti-inflammatory drugs (NSAIDs), acetaminophen, or COX-2 inhibitors alone fail to relieve pain (Altman et al., 2000). It is highly soluble in water. It is readily absorbed after oral administration. Its half life is about 6 hours (Grond and Sablotzki, 2004).

Diclofenac sodium (DS), a phenylacetic acid derivative, is an NSAID with a pK_a value of 4.0 (Figure-1.3). It exists in its acidic form in an acidic solution such as gastric juice, and is practically insoluble in water but soluble in intestinal fluid (Sheu et al., 1992). It is rapidly absorbed when given orally. It is used for the management of pain and inflammation in various musculoskeletal and joint disorders. Its plasma half life is about 1 to 2 hours. Its usual oral dose is 75 to 150 mg daily in divided doses (Fowler 1983).

Ethylcellulose (EC, Figure-1.4) with complete ethoxyl substitution (DS=3) is $C_{12}H_{23}O_6(C_{12}H_{22}O_5)_nC_{12}H_{23}O_6$ where "n" can vary to provide a wide variety of molecular weights. Ethylcellulose, an ethyl ether of cellulose, is a long chain polymer of β-anhydroglucose units joined together by acetal linkages. It is generally considered as a nontoxic, biocompatible and non-biodegradable polymer. These characteristics are the reasons of its extensive selection for the development of oral dosage forms, especially sustained release formulations. This is the reason why EC is extensively used for the development of oral multi-unit dosage forms (i.e. microparticles). EC coated microparticles have also demonstrated their capability to absorb pressure and therefore save the coating from fracture during tablet manufacturing process. This process involves the conversion of multi-unit system into a single unit dosage form by compression. This single unit system disintegrates slowly into sub-units when exposed to dissolution process (Rowe et al. 2003).

Some authors microencapsulated salbutamol sulphate using various polymers with thermal change and solvent evaporation techniques and studied the dissolution profiles of designed microcapsules. But no one has elaborated whether salbutamol sulphate is chemically stable and intact or not after its microencapsulation into ethylcellulose and none of them characterized morphology, rheological properties, FTIR spectroscopy, X-Ray diffractometry and thermal analysis of prepared microcapsules. Thus the objective of present work was to encapsulate salbutamol sulpahte (SS) into ethylcellulose (EC) microshells by different techniques i.e. coacervation thermal change (Yazan et al., 1995), solvent evaporation (Amperiadou

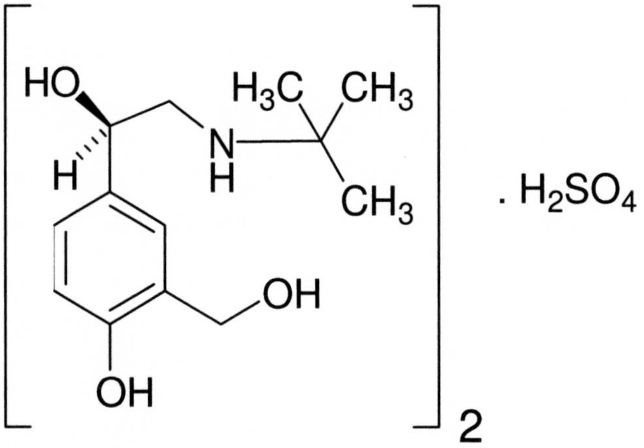

Figure 1.1: Chemical structure of Salbutamol sulphate

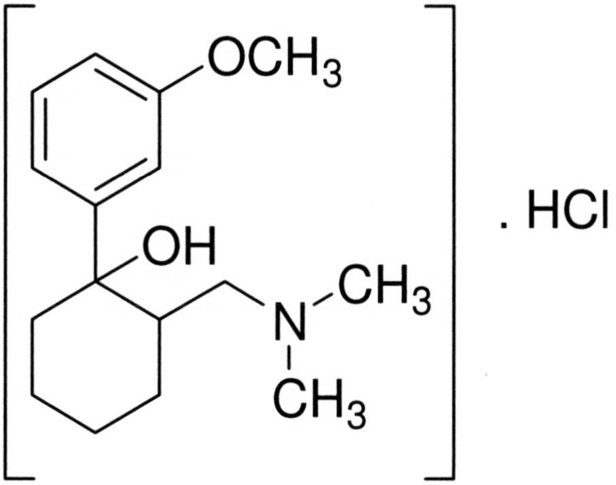

Figure 1.2: Chemical structure of Tramadol hydrochloride

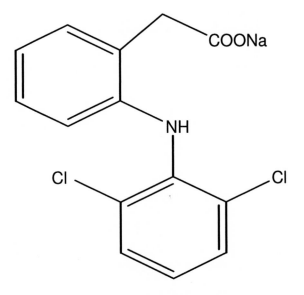

Figure 1.3: Chemical structure of Diclofenac sodium

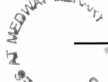

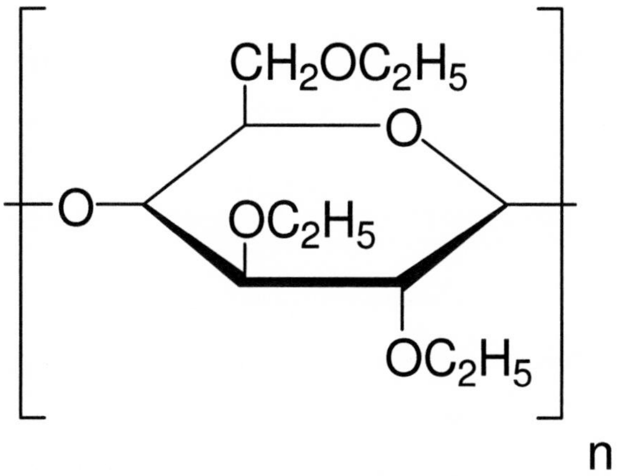

Figure 1.4: Chemical structure of Ethylcellulose

and Georgarakis, 1995; Erden and Celebi, 1996) and coacervation non-solvent addition (present research) and compared the designed microcapsules by applying various statistical, mathematical and analytical tools.

Tramadol hydrochloride has been microencapsulated into ethyl cellulose by spray drying and into polyhydroxybutyrate by solvent evaporation (Zhang et al., 2000; Salman et al., 2003). Literature also narrates few citations about microencapsulation of diclofenac sodium using different techniques (Sajeev et al., 2002; Biju et al., 2004). None of those, however, described characterization of microparticles using micromeritics, scanning electron microscope, FTIR, thermal analysis and X-ray diffractometry. Moreover, no record was found for the microencapsulation of diclofenac sodium with non solvent addition phase separation method. So keeping in mind the literature and pharmacokinetic data of DS, its microparticles with ethylcellulose were prepared and characterized. The aim of the present work was to construct a comparative study of SS, TH and DS formulations (microcapsules and tabletted microcapsules). Non-solvent addition coacervation was the microencapsulation technique used to produce microcapsules of these drugs.

We developed a RP-HPLC method for the quantitation of SS from human plasma for the comparison of developed formulation with that of the marketed formulation. This work is a part of the sustained release microencapsulated formulation development of SS and its pharmacokinetic evaluation in human. According to literature, several analytical methods have been developed for SS determination in the dosage forms and biofluids (Saleh et al., 2000, Sutariya et al., 2006, Forsdahl and Gmeiner, 2004, Qin et al., 2003).

In this context, we were interested to develop sensitive and specific HPLC method with FLD for the quantitative assay of SS in human plasma after LLE and the application of the method to a preliminary pharmacokinetic study in human. In order to optimize the separation, different chromatographic conditions were also studied and are described in this report.

FDA has developed a regulatory guidance for both immediate- and modified-release dosage forms to reduce the requirement of bioavailability studies as part of the formulation design and optimization. Increased development of modified-release dosage forms necessitates investigating the broader aspects of in vitro-in vivo correlation (IVIVC). If a class I drug is microencapsulated and converted into a slow release multi-unit dosage form in which the release profile controls the rate of absorption, and the solubility and permeability of the drug is site independent, an IVIVC is expected, otherwise limited or no correlations. In this continuity, present research also involves the development of an IVIVC for tabletted microcapsules of a water soluble drug (salbutamol sulphate) (Emami, 2006; Nefedova et al., 2005).

In present study, SS-EC microparticles prepared by non-solvent addition-phase separation varying EC ratio were tabletted and evaluated by various mathematical, statistical and analytical approaches followed by the development of IVIVC.

Literature

Review

2. LITERATURE REVIEW

2.1. Sustained Release Dosage Forms

Pharmaceutical formulations involve aqueous solutions, powders, dispersion concentrates, sustained release formulations, dry flowables and others. A rapidly increasing importance is observed in the development of sustained-release formulations of different drugs in present era of pharmaceutical technology. Sustained-release formulations are the dosage forms which allow slow dissolution and release of drug with respect to time. Sustained-release formulations have following advantages over immediate-release formulations:

1. Uniform drug level in blood.

2. Improvement in patient compliance.

3. Decrease in drug accumulation in stomach.

4. Extension in duration of activity for an equal level of active moiety.

5. Optimization of drug therapy.

6. Less chances of dose-related side effects.

7. Increase in drug efficacy.

8. Decrease in dosing frequency.

Development of sustained release formulation of an active moiety is strongly encouraged if it exhibits following characteristics:

1. Active moiety having short biological life.

2. Active moiety having broad therapeutic window.

3. Active moiety having relation between its pharmacological activity and blood levels.

4. Active moiety whose absorption occurs by passive transport.

The development of a sustained-release solid formulation involves the embedment of active moiety into some insoluble matrix e.g. ethylcellulse, eudragit etc. Whereas the release of drug from such formulations occurs through channels in the matrix following some suitable mechanism i.e. erosion, diffusion etc. Matrix tablets and tabletted microcapsules are two types of sustained-release solid formulations. In the present study, drug-polymer microcapsules were prepared by various microencapsulation techniques and then compressed into tablets to produce a sustained-release matrix.

2.2. Microencapsulation

2.2.1. What is Microencapsulation?

Microencapsulation is a coating process involving uniform deposition of some insoluble material (coat) around tiny active moieties (core) to produce microparticles for efficient applications. There is a wide range of coating (Resins, polysccharides, proteins, polymers, lipids and others) and core materials (foods, drugs, flavors and others, Table 2.1).

2.2.2. Objectives of Microencapsulation

Following are some important objectives of microencapsulation:

1. To develop and achieve the advantages of sustained release formulations.

2. To improve stability of some active moiety.

3. To mask bitter taste of active moiety.

4. To enhance drug absorption and thus decrease unwanted effects i.e. gastric irritation.

2.2.3. Polymer Used for Microencapsulation

On the basis of biogradability, polymers can be classified into following two categories:

Table 2.1 Previously Encapsulated Materials

• Acids	• Flame retardants	• Peroxides
• Activated carbons	• Flavors	• Pesticides
• Active metals	• Food ingredients	• Pharmaceuticals
• Adhesives	• Fuels	• Phase-change
• Alcohols	• Fumigants	materials
• Aldehydes	• Fungi	• Phenols
• Amines	• Fungicides	• Photographic
• Amino acids	• Hydrocarbons	agents
• Animal feed	• Indicators	• Pigments
ingredients	• Inks	• Proteins
• Antibiotics	• Inorganic salts	• Radioprotectors
• Antibodies	• Ion-exchange resins	• Reflective products
• Antioxidants	• Liquid	• Resin-curing
• Antiseptics	hydrocarbons	agents
• Aqueous solutions	• Lubricant additives	• Retinoids
• Bacteria	• Monomers	• Salts
• Biocells	• Oils	• Sealants
• Bleaches	• Organometallic	• Solvents
• Catalysts	compounds	• Sterilants
• Chemiluminescent	• Oxidizers	• Steroids
materials	• Paints	• Sweeteners
• Corrosion inhibitors	• Peptides	• Vaccine adjuvants
• Deodorants	• Perfumes	• Viruses
• Dyes	• Enzymes	• Vitamins

1. Biodegradable polymers

2. Non-biodegradable polymers

Ethylcellulose is a non-biodegradable polymer. Ethyl cellulose (a non-ionic ethyl ether of cellulose) is a derivative of cellulose in which some of the hydroxyl groups on the repeating glucose units are converted into ethyl ether groups. It contains not less than 44% and not more than 51% of ethoxy groups, calculated on dried basis. The number of ethyl groups can vary depending on the manufacture.

It is a white to light tan odorless powder whose melting point and specific density ranges are 240-255°C and 1.07-1.18, respectively. It is insoluble in water but soluble in a wide range of organic solvents. When water-soluble binders cannot be used, ethyl cellulose is often the polymer of choice. They are classified into a range of polymer viscosities for different applications.

Following are main applications of ethylcellulose:

1. Ethylcellulose is utilized for microencapsulation of various pharmaceuticals to stabilize them against active interactions, hydrolysis and oxidation.

2. It is also employed for tablet coating to impart sustained release to film coatings.

3. It is used as a tablet binder to impart plastic flow properties to particles. It is also suitable for direct compression, injection, molding and melt extrusion.

4. It is indicated for flavor masking to improve their taste through suppression of strong flavors.

Ethylcellulose is, therefore, used in pharmaceutical industries in large amounts. This is the reason why it is used in the present study.

2.2.4. Microencapsulation Techniques

2.2.4.1. Physical Methods

Physical methods for microencapsulation include pan coating, air suspension coating, centrifugal extrusion, vibrational nozzle, spray drying, spray chilling, rotary disk atomization, fluid bed coating, stationary nozzle coextrusion and submerged nozzle coextrusion (Benita, 2006).

2.2.4.2. Chemical Methods

Chemical methods for microencapsulation include interfacial polymerization, in-situ polymerization, matrix polymerization, phase separation, solvent evaporation, solvent extraction, nanoencapsulation, coacervation and liposome technology (Benita, 2006). In the present research work, coacervation (non-solvent addition and thermal change) and solvent evaporation techniques were adopted to microencapsulate drugs. Literature provides some data on microencapsulation of salbutamol sulphate by thermal coacervation and solvent evaporation and others. No study is found in literature about microencapsulation of salbutamol sulphate by non-solvent addition. Therefore, this technique was investigated to encapsulate salbutamol sulphate into ethylcellulose in the present project. The microcapsules, prepared by all these three techniques, were evaluated by various in-vitro analytical tests which were not performed by previous researchers.

2.2.4.2.1. Microencapsulation of Salbutamol Sulphate by Supercritical Precipitation

Al Frayh et al. (2008) elaborated that β2-agonists are extensively used to combat bronchial problems i.e. acute asthma etc. and still salbutamol is the most frequently prescribed drug in this class. That is why this drug is selected as a model in this study. Sustained release formulations of salbutamol sulphate have been developed by following different researchers using microencapsulation techniques.

Najafabadi et al. (2005) precipitated salbutamol sulphate (SS) by supercritical carbon dioxide (SC-CO2) using a home-made system at two different pressures. A mixture of drug and methanol was prepared and sprayed into SC fluid. Methanol was extracted by SC-CO_2 resulting in the formation of microparticles. The shape, size and FTIR analysis of formulated microparticles was also determined. Microparticles showed a wide range of size. Flak- and needle-shaped microparticles were observed. Flake-shaped microparticles were smaller in size than needle-shaped. The size distribution of processed material was narrower than unprocessed. It was evident from FTIR spectra that present technique has no significant effect on the chemical nature of drug.

2.2.4.2.2. Microencapsulation of Salbutamol Sulphate by Thermal Change

Yazan et al. (1995) wrote that salbutamol sulphate is a β_2-adrenergic agonist. Due to its short plasma half life, it was microencapsulated using ethylcellulose to develop sustained release formulation. Same amounts of drug and polymer were employed. Dissolution study of prepared microcapsules, pure drug, tabletted microcapsules and a marketed tablet was conducted. Microencapsulated formulations exhibited a slow release of drug. The specific surface area of microencapsulated salbutamol sulpahte was comparatively less than that of its pure state. The $t_{50\%}$ for microcapsules and tabletted microcapsules was 90 and 15 minutes, respectively.

Bhanja and Pal (1989) used a mixture of polyacrylic resin and eudragit RS 100 to microencapsulate salbutamol sulphate. They analyzed the release profiles by applying various kinetic models. The best fit kinetic model was higuchi model. They also calculated diffusivity rate constant and diffusion constant using Baker-Lonsdale technique at pH 1.2.

2.2.4.2.3. Microencapsulation of Salbutamol Sulphate by Solvent Evaporation

Pachuau et al. (2008) developed combined sustained release formulation of microencapsulated salbutamol sulphate and theophylline with ethylcellulose using solvent evaporation technique. Tween 80 and cyclohexane were used as dispersing and hardening agents, respectively. Various analytical techniques i.e. X-ray diffractometry, differential scanning calorimetry, infra-red spectroscopy, entrapment efficiency characterization, micromeritics and dissolution (pH 7.4 Phosphate buffer as dissolution medium) were employed to reveal any chemical interaction between drugs, and drug & polymer. Spherical, free-flowing and white microspheres with good entrapment efficiency were obtained. No chemical interaction was observed between drug and polymer. Sustained release behavior of formulations was observed till eight hours.

Erden and Celebi (1996) used various grades of PLGA for the microencapsulation of salbutamol sulphate by multiple emulsion solvent evaporation technique following 2^3 factorial design. Microsphere size and encapsulation efficiency were selected as dependent variables. The independent variables were PVA concentration, gelatin amount and drug loading. Sustained release behavior of formulations was observed till eight hours with PLGA 75/25. Buffer solution with pH 7.4 at 37 °C was used as dissolution medium. The dissolution profiles consisted of two phases i.e. instantaneous rapid and a subsequent slow release phase.

Amperiadou and Georgarakis (1995) used ethylcellulose in various ratios to microencapsulate salbutamol sulphate by emulsion-solvent evaporation technique and analyzed the effect of various stirrers (magnet and propeller). They analyzed the release profiles by applying various kinetic models. The best fit kinetic model was first order and higuchi model. Tween 80, a dispersing agent, affected the size of microparticles and dissolution profile. The microencapsulation technique and drug:polymer ratio affected the dissolution profile, physical properties and percentage loading of microparticles.

2.2.4.2.5. Microencapsulation of Tramadol Hydrochloride

Zhang et al. (2000) applied a column technique to complex tramadol with a sulfonic acid cation-exchange resin. They used different viscosity grades of ethylcellulose as coating agent to microencapsulate tramadol-resin complexes by spray-drying technique. A definite and smooth surface of microparticles prepared by using low viscosity EC was observed with the help of a scanning electron microscope. A slow release of drug from microparticles prepared by using low viscosity grades (10, 20 and 45 cp) was observed as compared to EC 100 cp microparticles. In the presence of a plasticizer, low viscosity-grade EC exhibited slow release of drug while release profiles showed no effect of middle viscosity-grade EC. Three different plasticizers exhibited an identical influence. A wide variety of microparticles was achieved using various solvents of similar toxicity. Dichloromethane or ethyl acetate produced microparticle with a definite shape and low rate of drug release. Acetone produced microparticle with a definite shape and high rate of drug release. The aggregated microparticles were achieved when ethanol was used as solvent.

Acosta et al. (2003) used a mixture of alginate and chitosan for the microencapsulation of tramadol hydrochloride by two different methods. In one method, they pumped alginate into a mixture of chitosan and calcium chloride (Microparticle A). In another method, they pumped alginate into a mixture of calcium chloride and sodium chloride and then added to the solution of chitosan (Microparticle B). Both procedures produced spherical microparticles. Basic medium produced greater swelling to these microparticles than acidic. Dissolution study of the microparticles was carried out in simulated intestinal as well as simulated stomach medium. Sixty four and eighty six percent tramadol release was observed from microcapsules A and B, respectively after dissolution of 24 hours in simulated intestinal fluid. After fitting the data in korsmeyer model, anomalous mode of tramadol release was found.

2.2.4.2.6. Microencapsulation of Diclofenac Sodium

Murthy and Chowdary (2005) prepared diclofenac sodium-ethylcellulose microparticles by emulsion solvent evaporation technique using three different solvents i.e. ethyl acetate, dichloromethane and chloroform. Most sustained effect on drug release was observed by chloroform. Large, discrete, spherical and free-flowing microparticles were achieved from all the solvents. Tramadol contents, dissolution profiles, wall thickness, size, morphology and encapsulation efficiency of prepared microparticles was determined. The release profiles were best fit to first order model.

Biju et al. (2004) used ethylcellulose and cellulose acetate phthalate to prepare enteric microparticles of diclofenac sodium by wet granulation and heat change techniques. Microparticles were analyzed for their size, micromeritics, encapsulation efficiency, drug loading, drug-polymer interaction and release kinetics in simulated gastric fluid for initial two hours and simulated intestinal fluid for subsequent six hours. The optimum formulation consisted of ethylcellulose and cellulose acetate phthalate (1:1.5) which was further tested by in-vivo evaluation for ulcerogenicity as well as pharmacodynamic efficacy. It exhibited better anti-inflammatory activity than marketed formulation.

Kumbar et al. (2002) used three various cross-linking agents i.e. sulphuric acid, thermal treatment and glutaraldehyde to produce diclofenac-chitosan microparticles. Microencapsulation method involved the preparation of water-in-oil emulsion, addition of cross-linking agent in the water phase and soaking of the prepared microparticles in diclofenac sodium saturated solution. Microparticles were evaluated by scanning electron microscopy, x-ray diffractometry and FTIR spectroscopy. Dissolution study was carried out in 7.4 pH buffer solution. Microparticles were spherical. FTIR study proved that cross-linking of chitosan occurs at free amino group to form ionic bond. X-ray diffractometry evidenced that crystallinity of polymer increases enhanced after cross-linking. Drug loading efficiency was best for the microparticles prepared by sulphuric acid as cross-linking agent. Glutaraldehyde- and thermal treated-crosslinked microparticles exhibited a slow and fast drug release respectively.

Sajeev et al. (2002) formulated various ethylcellulose-diclofenac sodium microparticles by thermal change coacervation method and compressed these microparticles into sustained release oral tablets. Microparticles and tablets were evaluated for physical properties and dissolution profiles by paddle method in distilled water. Micropartciles were fine, spherical and free flowing. The release of drug sustained with increase in polymer concentration and wall thickness of microparticles. The physical properties of microparticles were evaluated according to compendial requirement. The release data was best fit to the zero order model. The rate of drug release was well correlated with polymer concentration in microparticles. The rate of drug release was well correlated with polymer concentration and tablet weight. Good stability and producibility was observed for all the formulations.

2.2.5. Mechanisms of Monitoring Drug Release

The mechanisms which monitor the release of drug from microcapsules are given below:

1. This category involves the release of drug in a delayed, controlled, sustained or targeted fashion.

2. This category involves the pulsatile, osmotic, thermal, pressure, enteric and pH-induced release of drug.

3. The release of drug induced by salt or by biodegradation is other mechanism of drug release.

4. This category involves the delivery of drug by pulmonary, implantable, oral, intranasal or injectable method (Benita, 2006, Banakar, 1992).

2.2.6. In-Vitro Evaluation of Microcapsules

Microcapsules can be analyzed using following various in-vitro analytical approaches i.e. determination of particle size, morphology study, drug release study, tablet hardness test, viscosity test, surface tension determination and Fourier transform infrared (FTIR). Nuclear magnetic resonance (NMR) spectroscopy, high performance liquid chromatographs (HPLC), differential scanning calorimeter (DSC), thermogravimetric analyzer (TGA), gas chromatograph/mass spectrometer (GC/MS) and ultraviolet-visible spectrophotometer are also used for the analysis of microparticles (Benita, 2006, Ohannesian, 2002).

2.2.7. In-Vivo Evaluation of Salbutamol Sulphate

2.2.7.1. Determination of salbutamol sulphate

Loden et al. (2008) analyzed salbutamol in Ventolin Depot tablets using a multiple-injection capillary zone electrophoresis method. Seven samples, three injections of each sample, were injected into the capillary and analyzed within a single run. Thus 21 injections were made in a row. 30 kV voltage was applied intermittently over the capillary to separate injected sample plugs from background electrolyte plugs. Partial electrophoresis was applied for 10.50 and 2.35 min to separate sample sets and samples in each set, respectively. After the last injection, all the applied samples were subjected to electrophoresis for a time period corresponding to that in conventional single-injection CZE. Firstly, accuracy, precision, linearity and robustness were determined to validate the method and then analyzed salbutamol in 15 Ventolin Depot tablets, each containing 8 mg salbutamol. The analysis of 15 tablet revealed that each tablet contained 7.8 mg salbutamol.

Sirichai and Khanatharana (2008) analyzed salbutamol, clenbuterol, fenoterol and procaterol simultaneously using a newly developed and validated capillary electrophoresis method attached with UV detector. A 32°C separation temperature, separation voltage 19 kV and 10 mmoll^{-1} borate buffer (pH 10.0) was applied to analyze the four drugs in dosage forms and human urine. No interfering peaks were observed. The detection limits were between 0.5 and 2.0 mgl^{-1} for these drugs. The calibration curve was constructed in a range of 2.0-30 mgl^{-1}. The correlation coefficient was greater than 0.996.

El-Gindy et al. (2007) showed that separation of the components of drug mixtures was carried out using spectrophotometeric methods previously. Currently HPLC is being under use for this purpose. In its continuity, the project was designed to resolve the components of various mixtures of drugs. In this study, two mixtures of drugs i.e. mixture A and mixture B were involved. Mixture A consisted of guaiphenesine, salbutamol sulfate (SL), methylparaben (MP) and propylparaben (PP) where as mixture B consisted of acephylline piperazine (AC), bromhexine hydrochloride (BX), methylparaben (MP) and propylparaben (PP). HPLC conditions for mixture A were as; reverse phase C18 column, ambient temperature conditions, UV detector operated at 243 nm and mobile phase consisting of 0.05 M KH$_2$PO$_4$ and acetonitrile (60 : 40, v/v) where as mobile phase containing 0.05 M KH$_2$PO$_4$ and acetonitrile (50 : 50, v/v) with pH 3 (50:50, v/v) and UV detector was operated at 245 nm. This method was accurate, linear, precise, specific and accurate. This method can therefore easily be applied for the screening of various mixtures of drugs.

Sherri et al. (2007) introduced a RP-enantioselective liquid chromatography–tandem mass spectrometry (HPLC-MS-MS) method. They analyzed waste water and determined ratio of enantiomers as well as drug amount. A stationary phase, Chirobiotic V, was used to detect enantiomers of atenolol, metoprolol, nadolol, pindolol, propranolol, sotalol, citalopram, fluoxetine, and salbutamol. The mean percentage recovery was eighty six percent in influent and seventy eight percent in effluent. The lowest limit of detection was 0.2-7.5 ng/L. Present study showed improved enumeration for all these drugs in waste-waters. The variation in EF by treatment showed biologically mediated stereoselective procedures which were possibly occurring during waste-water treatment.

Erram et al. (2006) conducted a study for the development and validation of a reverse-phase HPLC method attached with a UV-detector operated at 225 nm. This method was used for the detection of salbutamol sulphate and its 6 relevant substances. The specifications of column used were YMC phenyl column (250 mm x 4.6mm ID, 5 μm at ambient conditions. The mobile phase consisted of 25 mM monobasic potassium phosphate (pH 3.0) and methanol (95:5, v/v), delivered at 1.5 mL/min. An external standard was employed to quantify salbutamol. This method determined salbutamol and its 6 relevant substances efficiently on the basis of percent area. One of the relevant substances, bis-ether salbutamol, was separated on the basis of its hydrophilic nature. Another relevant substance, salbutamol aldehyde, was also separated. The lowest limit of detection and quantitation for salbutamol and its 6 relevant substances was 0.01 and 0.21% of the assay concentration of 0.3 mg/mL as salbutamol base. The calibration curve for salbutamol and the relevant substances was linear over 50-150% and 0.05-0.5% of the active label claim. The chromatograms showed no interfering peaks. This method showed good accuracy, precision, ruggedness, robustness, linearity and specificity.

Jianli et al. (2006) developed a liquid chromatography–electrospray ionization-mass spectrometry (LC–ESI-MS) with good sensitivity and specificity for the determination of salbutamol in human urine using nadolol as the internal standard. Glucuronidase was used to hydrolyze urine samples. Then these samples are extracted using solid phase extraction process. An Agilent Zorbax SB-C18 column was used in this study. The mobile phase consisted of 0.01 M ammonium formate buffer (pH 3.5)–acetonitrile (85:15, v/v). The quantification of samples was accomplished using positive electrospray. Salbutamol and nadolol were determined by m/z 166 and m/z 310. The calibration curve was constructed over a concentration range of 10-2000 ng/ml. The lowest limit of detection was found to be ten monograms per milliliter. The intra- and inter-run precision was < 7.3% while accuracy was within ± 2.6%. The excretion plots of salbutamol were constructed using this method.

Sutariya et al. (2006) quantified salbutamol sulphate in rabbit plasma using a new RP-HPLC-UV (λ = 276 nm) method. Analytical column (4.6 × 250 mm) C18 was used. Mobile phase (H_2O : CH_3OH : Acetonitrile, 70 : 20 : 10 V/V) was run at 1.2 ml/min. This method showed good simplicity, specificity, precision and accuracy. Chloramphenicol was used as internal standard. Five milliliter of 0.1 M di-(2-ethylhexyl) phosphate (DEHP) in chloroform was added to extract drug and internal standard followed by the addition of chloroform layer to 0.5 M HCl. A sufficient quantity of HCl layer was injected to HPLC. No interfering peaks were observed. The retention time was 3.0 and 15.4 min for salbutamol sulphate and chloramphenicol.

The standard curve was linear between 100 to 1500 ng/ml whose coefficient of determination was equal to 0.992. The extraction efficiency was more than eighty percent. The lowest limit of quantification was 100 ng/ml. The percent recovery of drug was between 99-102%. The interday- and intraday-coefficient of variation ranges were 1.9-6.2% and 1.1-8.9%, respectively. This method was applied to study in-vivo kinetics of salbutamol sulphate when administered as different oral formulations to rabbits.

Jin et al. (2005) developed an ion chromatography method with direct conductivity detection without chemical suppression for the determination of salbutamol pharmacokinetics. The mobile phase was 2 mM/L HNO3 with 6% acetonitrile (v/v). Atenolol was used as internal standard. The calibration curve was linear over a concentration range of 3 to 1000 ng/ml with a coefficient of determination equal to 0.996. The lowest limit of detection of salbutamol was 1 ng/ml. Eight milligram salbutamol was given to eighteen human subjects followed by the collection of blood samples and analysis of data to calculate various noncompartmental pharmacokinetic parameters for salbutamol.

Halabi et al. (2004) determined, quantified, screened and confirmed the enantiomers of salbutamol using a rapid and validated chiral HPLC method with good specificity and reliability. Salbutamol sulphate was separated from known impurities using a set of optimum chiral HPLC conditions.

Isabel and Moises (2004) presented a flow-injection method for the detection of salbutamol. In the presence of hexacyanoferrate (III) in alkaline medium, they condensed salbutamol with 4-aminoantipyrine and obtained a coloured quinoneimide whose absorption spectra was obtained by operating spectrophotometer at 500 nm. The sequential simplex method was used to optimize the values of 4 variables which were studied in univariant way. They developed a new methodology for the determination of salbutamol sulphate in marketed oral solutions as well as tablets. This validated method was compared with the reference compendial method. The precision of both methods was similar to each other. The standard curve was linear over a range of zero to 74.1 mg/L whose coefficient of determination was equal to 0.9999. The analysis of seventy five samples per hour was possible using this method.

Rosa et al. (2000) conducted this study to provide a base for the differentiation between the IOC authorized use (inhaled) and the IOC prohibited use (oral) of salbutamol. It involved the urine analysis to enumerate the level of nonconjugated enantiomers of salbutamol. According to this study, 5 doses of 4 mg or 2 doses of 100 µg salbutamol were given to asthmatic and non-asthmatic human subjects. After dosing, urine samples were collected at pre-determined time points. Similarly, maximum inhaled salbutamol doses (1600 µg in 24 h, 800 µg being in the last 4 h) were also given to the persons suffering from exercise-induced asthma. Urine samples were also collected from these subjects at pre-determined time points. The analysis of these samples was carried out to elaborate the quantity of salbutamol and percentage of S- and R-enantiomers. The data could be classified in to two categories on the basis of differentiation factor; inhaled and oral. According to confirmation criteria, oral classified as inhaled rate was 11.8% where as inhaled classified as oral rate was nil. Free salbutamol amount was less than 500 µg/L determined by gas chromatography-mass spectrometry. Salbutamol and its conjugate sulphate level was greater than 1400 µg/L determined by ELISA.

2.2.7.2. Pharmacokinetics Studies of Salbutamol sulphate

Al Frayh et al. (2008) revealed that salbutamol is still one of the most leading prescribed drugs for the treatment of asthma. They prepared a random, two doses

(100, 200μg of Butalin and ventolin inhalers), open label, multicenter and cross-over study design to study pharmacokinetics of salbutamol sulphate in 89 patients (62% were male) with mild and moderate asthma states for four days. The forced expiratory volume (FEV) and peak expiratory flow (PEF) were calculated at different time points. The two tested formulations showed significant similarity with respect to their FEV and PEF values. Both drugs showed significantly similar strength, start and duration of activity. It reveals that both of the formulations were bioequivalent.

Hongfei et al. (2007) used beagle dogs to determine pharmacokinetics of the salbutamol sulfate pulsatile-release capsules using HPLC method. The pharmacokinetic parameters of test and standard tablets were determined. It was concluded from the results that both formulations are bioequivalent.

Taha et al. (2004) studied bioequivalence of 3 suppository formulations of two milligram salbutamol sulphate using various bases i.e. Suppocire NA with 6% Eudispert, Witepsol H with 3% methylcellulose gel and Witepsol W25 with 3% methylcellulose gel. This 4 way crossover study involved 6 normal male human adults to whom these formulations were administered separately with a wash out period of one week between each sampling. The rate and extent of absorption of drug from the suppositories and two milligram tablets was determined. Five milliliter blood samples were drawn from veins at different time points. It was concluded from the study that Suppocire NA with 6% Eudispert and Witepsol W25 with 3% methylcellulose gel improved salbutamol sulphate bioavailability which was similar to that of oral tablets. Present study also revealed that rectal administration is a good substitute of orally administered salbutamol sulphate tablets.

Hindle et al. (2003) elaborated that new research should be made on new drug delivery devices i.e. dry powder inhaler (DPI) and they should be preferred over previously adopted drug delivery devices i.e. metered dose inhaler (MDI). In this study, urine samples were analyzed to find the rate and extent of salbutamol absorption in lungs after delivery using DPI (Innovata) and MDI (Ventolin) following a randomized, double-blind, two way crossover study design in ten human subjects. Urine was also analyzed to find the quantity of salbutamol and its conjugated metabolite to determine its relative bioavailability of salbutamol to the body. The results showed that delivery of salbutamol is in higher amount by DPI than that of MDI. It approves the aim of more research in the field of DPI. The inhalation drug delivery systems can be differentiated.

Boulton and Fawcett (1996) described that salbutamol is a racemate with β_2-agonistic activity. Its bronchodilation activity mainly depends upon R-enantiomer, slightly on S-enantiomer. Salbutamol is metabolized largely in liver and excreted in urine. This study was conducted to find out enantiomeric pharmacokinetics of salbutamol after its intravenous (1.6 mg) and oral (4 mg) doses to 7 healthy male human volunteers. Plasma samples were extracted by solid phase and then injected into chiral HPLC for analysis. After intravenous dosing of salbutamol, the ratio of R/S enantiomers of salbutamol in urine and blood samples was one soon after drug administration and 0.66 after eight hours. After oral dosing of salbutamol, the ratio of R/S enantiomers of salbutamol in urine and blood samples was 0.3 over eight hours. The clearance rate, terminal half life and amount of drug eliminated in urine after oral administration were significantly differed from that of oral. After oral administration, it was also found that metabolism of R-enantiomer of salbutamol was quicker than that of S-enantiomer due to which low bioavailability of R-enantiomer was observed.

Morgan et al. (1986) administered salbutamol intravenously and orally to ten normal human subjects to elaborate pharmacokinetics of salbutamol and its conjugated metabolite. The elimination of drug via urine was greater after its intravenous dosing. The sulphate conjugate detected was an indication of first pass effect of this drug through the wall of intestine. A directly proportional relationship was observed between the rate of heart beat and salbutamol level in human plasma.

2.2.8. Biowaiver Studies

2.2.8.1. Introduction of biowaiver studies

Drugs undergo various changes after their administration. These changes are described by bioavailability which reports the rate and extent of entrance of a drug into blood flow after its absorption (Rowland and Tozer, 1995; Barret, 2004). Drug bioavailability is affected by following various factors: solubility, particle size, dosage form variables etc. In poor regions of the world, the launching of low price drug products with good quality has ever been required. In the early era of bioavailability, it was narrated that two products, having same active agent in same amount, may vary from each other in regard of their efficacy and efficiency, thus needing their bioequivalence studies. This problem is serious with low therapeutic range drugs e.g. digoxin. Many guidelines regarding bioavailability and bioequivalence of new drug products have been presented in 1977, 1995, 1997, 2000 and 2007 by Food and Drug Administration authority and other scientists. A decreased need of in vivo bioequivalence studies due to in-vitro in-vivo correlation (IVIVC) and BCS biowaiver guidelines is observed. This study has not been conducted as frequently as was imagined. However, The World Health Organization (WHO) has actively utilized BCS biowaivers (WHO, 2006).

New pharmaceutical products can be formulated on the basis of IVIVC and BCS biowaiver guidelines. IVIVC is classified into level A, B and C (Table 2.2 and 2.3). Level A IVIVC development needs a discriminative dissolution method which can act as a surrogate of in-vivo bioequivalence studies. A discriminative dissolution method is developed under various controlled conditions keeping in mind the gastrointestinal physiology (Dressman et al., 1998). The gastrointestinal tract (GIT) exhibits a variety of conditions of various variables such as pH, lumen fluid volumes, contents, etc. The pH range of empty and fed stomach fluid is 1.4-2.1 and 3-7 (Dressman et al., 1990; Dressman et al., 1998). The pH range of fasting and fed small intestine fluid is 4.4 to 8.0 (Gray and Dressman, 1996). The pH of small intestine is also affected by the salts (solubility factor) excreted by liver (Dressman et al., 1998). The mean fluid volume in fasting stomach, jejunum and ileum is 30, 130 and 340 ml (Wilson and Washington, 1989; Dressman et al., 1998; Schiller et al., 2005; Dillard et al., 1965). Drug solubility in GIT is also affected by the duration of drug stay and mixing (Dressman et al, 1998; Davis et al., 1986; Yu et al., 1996). The absorption of highly soluble pharmaceutical agents from their immediate release dosage forms occurs mainly from the upper intestine. The absorption of poorly soluble and poorly permeable pharmaceutical agents from their immediate release dosage forms occurs mainly from the small intestine and colon in slow speed. Similarly, slow absorption of drugs from modified release dosage forms occur in small intestine and colon. All these variables affect the performance of drug (Dokoumetzidis and Macheras, 2006). The movement and contents of gastrointestinal fluids are also needed to be substituted in in-vitro dissolution evaluation (Dressman et al., 1998; Dokoumetzidis and Macheras, 2006; Dressman, 2001; Dressman, 2007). In short, a discriminative dissolution medium is necessary for surrogative studies.

2.2.8.2. Modified-release formulations

The development of modified-release dosage forms of rapidly excreted drugs is very urgent because an optimum therapeutic drug concentration should be maintained in

Table 2.2: The Biopharmaceutical Classification System

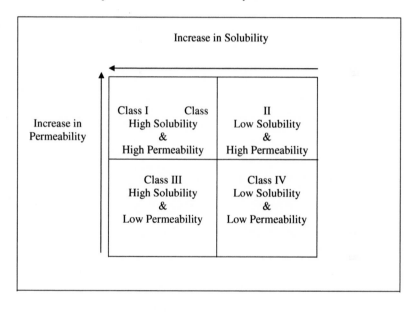

Table 2.3: Criteria for biowaiver studies

Eligibility for BCS Based Biowaiver Differs Between FDA, CPMP (EU) and WHO			
	FDA 2000	*CPMP (EU) NFG 2001*	***WHO 2005***
High Solubility	pH 1 to 7.5 Highest tablet strength	pH 1 to 6.8 Highest tablet strength	pH 1.2 to 6.8 Highest dose
High Permeability (f_a)	Equal to and less than 90%	Linear/complete Absorption	Less than 85%
Dissolution	Equal to and less than 85% pH 1, 4.5, 6.8 50 rpm (paddle) 100 rpm (basket)	Equal to and less than 85% pH 1, 4.5, 6.8 Equipment not specified	Equal to and less than 85% pH 1, 4.5, 6.8 75 rpm (paddle) 100 rpm (basket)

the body (Rowland and Tozer, 1995). The modified-release dosage forms may be microencapsulated, floating, mucoadhesive etc. (Davis, 2005; Lennernas and Abrahamsson, 2004; Thombre, 2005). Various drugs belonging to various BCS classes show different absorption potentials (Ungell et al., 1998).

2.2.8.3. Uses of in-vitro in-vivo correlation

1. To design a discriminative dissolution method that can serve as a substitute of in-vivo bioavailability or bioequivalence evaluation.

2. To make post-marketed changes

2.2.8.4. Establishment of in-vitro in-vivo correlation

According to FDA guidelines 1997, 2 or 3 formulations are required and evaluated to develop level A IVIVC model between in-vitro and in-vivo data (FDA guidance, 1997). In first step of level A IVIVC development, the data is converted into cumulative absorbed drug (%) by any of the following approaches: such as Wagner-Nelson and Loo-Riegelman, or model independent procedures (Wagner and Nelson, 1964; Loo and Riegelman, 1968; Cutler, 1978; Veng-Pedersen, 1992). For one- and two-compartment model, Wagner-Nelson and Loo-Riegelman method is applied.

2.2.8.5. In-vitro in-vivo correlation

Valenzuela et al. (2006) elaborated the exact absorption mechanism of salbutamol sulphate using small intestine of rats, followed by the development of a semi-physiological population pharmacokinetic model. Various concentrations of salbutamol sulphate (0.15 to 18 mM) were applied to study its absorption by different in-situ methods. Salbutamol sulphate (0.29 mM) was co-administered with verapamil (10 and 20 mM), grapefruit juice and sodium azide (NaN$_3$) (0.3, 3 and 6 mM). The data obtained was analyzed using various pharmacokinetic models i.e. parametric and non-parametric bootstrap analyses. By applying this model, an instantaneous equilibrium of salbutamol sulphate was observed between intestinal lumen and enterocyte which was best explained by simultaneous passive diffusion, active absorption and active capacity-limited efflux. An improved absorption of salbutamol sulphate was observed in the presence of NaN_3, grapefruit juice and verapamil.

Kuksal et al. (2006) used eudragit RLPO and RSPO alone or in combination with ethyl cellulose to prepare sustained release matrix tablets of zidovudine followed by their characterization using scanning electron microscopy and dissolution. The formulated tablets were compared to the marketed conventional tablets by in-vitro and in-vivo techniques. The tablet formulation prepared with any of the eudragit alone controlled the release of drug until 6th hour. The tablet formulation prepared with any of the eudragit combined with ethylcellulose controlled the release of drug until 12th hour. The application of Korsmeyer-Peppas model to the dissolution data evidenced that the release of drug from the formulated tablets was a combination of diffusion and erosion. The formulation prepared with eudragit-ethylcellulose combination was tested by in-vivo evaluation using rabbits. It was concluded from the results that formulated slow release zidovudine tablets could show good performance therapeutically.

Emami (2006) stated that this review paper includes FDA guidelines, data required for the development, characterization and validation of an IVIVC and dissolution requirements on the basis of biopharmaceutics classification systems (BCS). This paper also describes the knowledge of in-vitro and in-vivo behaviour and their correlation (IVIVC) of a formulation is necessary for its development and biopharmaceutics studies. Therefore, a requirement is still present to correlate in-vitro data with in-vivo results which enhance formulation quality, reduce cost and reduce the time required for drug development. A progressive trend in the development of

IVIVC is a good sign for pharmaceutical industry. The most important usefulness of IVIVC development is the decreased need of human volunteers for the bioavailability studies and bioequivalence evaluations which is the base of biowaiver study or surrogative study. The biowaiver study targets the development of a discriminative dissolution method that can act as a substitute of in-vivo studies. IVIVC has got a high level importance during the scale-up, post-approval changes and the development of modified release dosage forms. This paper also describes the validation of IVIVC that involves internal and external validation. It also concludes that the principles for conventional oral dosage forms needed for IVIVC are similar to that of non-oral and modified-release dosage forms.

Grass and Sinko (2002) showed the importance of drug selection equivalent to drug discovery and development. The predictive, good quality, quick and correlative pharmacokinetic models are needed for an efficient drug selection. Currently, no reliable system is available that can be useful for the correct prediction of drug attitude in human. Therefore, typical tools are in use to decide about the behavior of drug in body until its clinical trial. However, pharmacokinetics should be characterized accurately and rapidly using some suitable software due to the current advancement in genomics and proteomics.

2.9. Salbutamol Sulphate

Salbutamol is a short acting β_2-adrenergic agonist with less effect on β_1-adrenoceptors of cardiac muscles. It is used for the treatment of mild to severe bronchoconstriction.

2.9.1. Formula of Salbutamol Sulphate

2.9.1.1. Molecular formula of salbutamol sulphate

The molecular formula of salbutamol sulphate is $(C_{13}H_{21}NO_3)_2H_2SO_4$ (USP-NF, 2004).

2.9.1.2. Molecular weight of salbutamol sulphate

The molecular weight of salbutamol sulphate is 576.7 g/mol (USP-NF, 2004).

2.9.1.3. Melting point of salbutamol sulphate

The melting point of salbutamol sulphate is 157-158°C (with decomposition) (USP-NF, 2004).

2.9.1.4. Description of salbutamol sulphate

It is white or almost white powder and odorless or almost odorless (USP-NF, 2004).

2.9.1.5. Solubility of salbutamol sulphate

Salbutamol sulphate is soluble in 4 parts of water; slightly soluble in ethanol (96%), chloroform and ether (USP-NF, 2004).

2.9.1.6. pH of salbutamol sulphate

A 5% solution of salbutamol sulphate in distilled water has a pH value of 4.3 (Ritschel and Kearns, 2004, USP-NF, 2004).

2.9.1.7. pKa values of salbutamol sulphate

Salbutamol has pKa values of 9.3 and 10.3 (Ritschel and Kearns, 2004).

2.9.1.8. Partition coefficient values of salbutamol sulphate

The distribution coefficient of salbutamol between 2 phases of octanol and water, as determined by HPLC, is log D=-0.5 at pH 7.42 at room temperature (Ritschel and Kearns, 2004).

2.9.1.9. Mechanism of action of salbutamol sulphate

Before discussion of mechanism of action of salbutamol sulphate, it seems necessary to discuss pathophysiology of asthma. Asthma is characterized by fluctuating airways obstruction, with a diurnal variation. This manifests as a triad of wheeze, cough and breathlessness. In allergic asthma, which is generally of early onset, extrinsic allergens produce a type I allergic reaction in atopic subjects (Figure 2.1 and 2.2). Type I reactions are associated with the presence of reaginic antibodies (IgE) on the surface of mast cells and probably other immune effector cells (eosinophils and lymphocytes).

Patients with non-allergic (late onset) asthma do not appear to be sensitive to any well-defined antigen, although infection (usually viral) often precipitates an attack. These acute inflammatory processes can ultimately lead to irreversible lung damage. Inflammatory mediators that have been implicated include histamine, serotonin, prostaglandin D_2, kinins and others. Increased parasympathetic tone also causes bronchoconstriction.

Salbutamol, a β_2-adrenergic agonist, occupies and stimulates β_2-adrenergic receptors resulting in the relaxation of bronchial smooth muscles. It is assumed that salbutamol stimulates adenylate cyclase that enhances cyclic adenosine monophosphate (cAMP) production through membrane-bound coupled G-proteins. It, subsequently, inhibits the release of mast cell mediators in the airways. Additionally, increased cAMP production increases the activity of cAMP-dependent protein kinase which ultimately inhibits the phosphorylation of myosin and lowers intracellular calcium concentration. A lowered intracellular calcium concentration causes the relaxation of bronchial smooth muscles (Figure 2.3) (Goodman & Gilman, 2006).

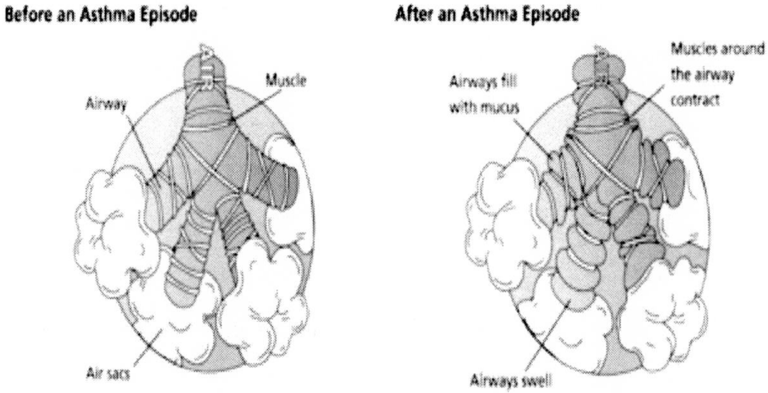

Before an Asthma Episode

Muscle

Airway

Air sacs

After an Asthma Episode

Muscles around the airway contract

Airways fill with mucus

Airways swell

Figure 2.1: Inflamed airways and bronchoconstriction in asthma. Airways narrowed as a result of the inflammatory response cause wheezing. (http://en.wikipedia.org/wiki/Asthma)

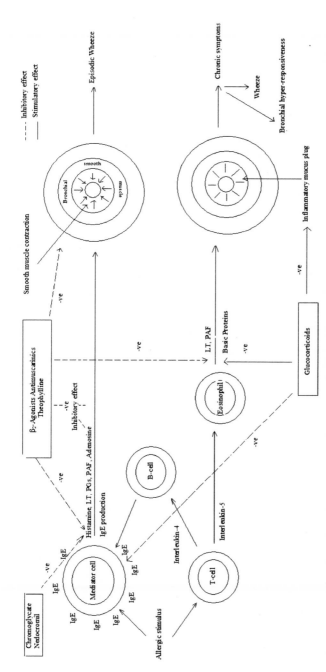

Figure 2.2: Pathophysiology of asthma and sites of drug action. PAF = Platelet-Activating Factor, LTs = Leukotrienes, PGs = Prostaglandins. (Courtesy from: J. M. Ritter, L. D. Lewis, T. G. K. Mant. A text book of clinical pharmacology. 4th Edition, 1999)

2.9.1.10. Pharmacokinetics of salbutamol sulphate

Salbutamol sulphate is readily absorbed from the gastrointestinal tract. Maximum plasma concentration achieves within 2.5 hours. Orally administered salbutamol sulphate undergoes pronounced first pass metabolism (50%) in the liver to form an inactive metabolite (sulphate conjugates, 4-O sulphate or phenolic sulphate) that is excreted in the urine along with unmetabolized salbutamol. 76% of an oral dose is eliminated over three days. Comparatively less salbutamol is excreted as sulphate conjugate after intravenous administration. Most (80%) of the dose administered by aerosol is swallowed so systemic absorption is low, but the inhaled fraction (10-20%) largely remains as free drug in the airways and does not appear to be metabolized in the lungs. The plasma half life is 4-6 hours. Salbutamol does not pass blood brain barrier (Ritter et al., 1999).

2.9.1.11. Pharmacological effects of salbutamol sulphate

The pharmacological effects produced by the use of salbutamol sulphate are following:

1. Relaxation of bronchial smooth muscles.
2. Inhibition of release of inflammatory mediators.
3. Enhanced mucocilliary clearance.
4. Relaxation of uterine smooth muscles.

(Ritter et al., 1999)

2.9.1.13. Uses of salbutamol sulphate

Salbutamol sulphate is suitable for following conditions:

1. Management and prevention of severe or unstable asthma
2. Chronic bronchitis
3. Emphysema

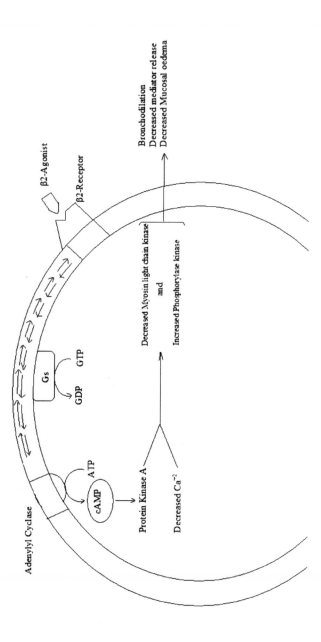

Figure 2.3: Membrane and intracellular events triggered when β2-agonists stimulate β2-receptors. Gs = stimulatying G-protein, GDP = guanosine diphosphate, GTP = guanosine triphosphate, cAMP = cyclic adenosine monophosphate.

4. Uncomplicated premature labour during the third trimester of pregnancy. (Martindale, 2002)

2.9.1.14. Dosage forms of salbutamol sulphate

Different dosage forms of salbutamol sulphate are available as given below:

Injection: Salbutamol sulphate equivalent to 0.5 mg salbutamol is present in 1 ml ampoule of its injection.

Syrup: Salbutamol sulphate equivalent to 2 mg salbutamol is present in 5 ml its syrup.

Sustained release tablets 4 mg / 8 mg contain salbutamol sulphate equivalent to 4 mg / 8 mg salbutamol.

Tablets 2 mg / 4 mg contain salbutamol sulphate equivalent to 2 mg / 4 mg salbutamol.

Inhaler: Each actuation of metered dose aerosol contains 100 μg salbutamol.

(Physician Desk Reference, 2001)

2.9.1.15. Dose of salbutamol sulphate

Injection: In severe bronchospasm and status asthmaticus, 8 μg/kg IV or SC is administered four hourly in adults and not recommended in children. In uncomplicated premature labour, 100-250 μg by IV infusion or IV injection or IM injection. The dose may be repeated according to the response of patient.

Tablets/Syrup: In bronchial problems, 2-4 mg salbutamol is given three or four times daily in adults and 1-2 mg three or four times daily in children of 2-12 years. Inhaler: In acute asthma or before exercise, 100-400 μg salbutamol is used in adults. The maintenance dose is 100-400 μg three to four times daily. Maximum dose is 1.6 mg/day. In episodic asthma or before exercise, 100-200 μg salbutamol is used in children. The maintenance dose is 100-200 μg three to four times daily. Maximum dose is 0.8 mg/day (Physician Desk Reference, 2001)

2.9.1.16. Adverse effects of salbutamol

The adverse effects produced by the use of salbutamol sulphate are following:

1. Arrhythmias

2. Palpitations

3. Muscle tremors

4. Hypokalaemia

5. Raised free fatty acid concentrations

6. Increased blood sugar

7. Tolerance of β_2-agonists

8. Hyperkinesis

9. Drowsiness

10. Agitation

11. Flushing

12. Allergic reaction

13. Indigestion

(Ritter et al., 1999)

2.9.1.17. Interaction of salbutamol sulphate with other drugs

Salbutamol sulphate should not be indicated with other sympathomimetic agents. Bronchodilation activity of salbutamol is inhibited by β-antagonists e.g. propranolol (Martindale, 2002).

2.9.1.18. Contra-indications of salbutamol sulphate

Salbutamol sulphate is not indicated in the patients with the history of hypersensitivity to any of its components (Martindale, 2002).

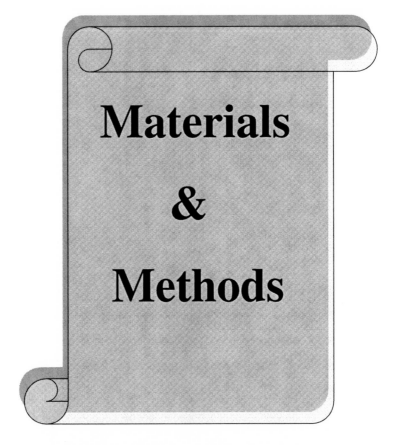

Formulation Development of Salbutamol by Microencapsulation, Its In-Vitro and In-Vivo Studies

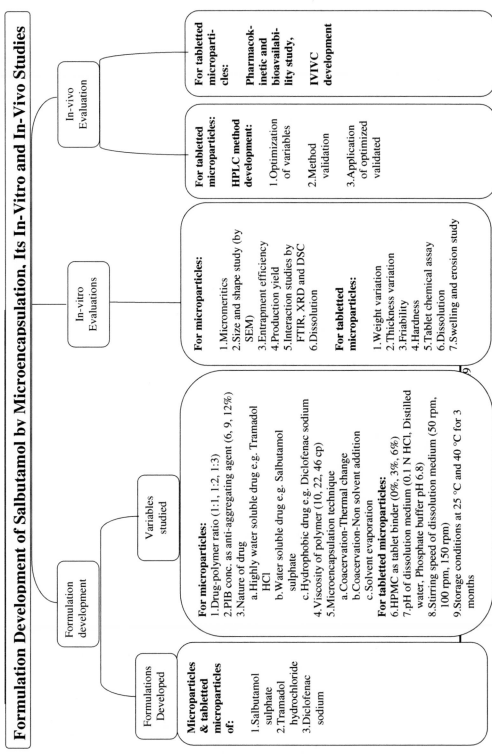

Formulation development

Formulations Developed

Microparticles & tabletted microparticles of:

1. Salbutamol sulphate
2. Tramadol hydrochloride
3. Diclofenac sodium

Variables studied

For microparticles:
1. Drug-polymer ratio (1:1, 1:2, 1:3)
2. PIB conc. as anti-aggregating agent (6, 9, 12%)
3. Nature of drug
   a. Highly water soluble drug e.g. Tramadol HCl
   b. Water soluble drug e.g. Salbutamol sulphate
   c. Hydrophobic drug e.g. Diclofenac sodium
4. Viscosity of polymer (10, 22, 46 cp)
5. Microencapsulation technique
   a. Coacervation-Thermal change
   b. Coacervation-Non solvent addition
   c. Solvent evaporation

For tabletted microparticles:
6. HPMC as tablet binder (0%, 3%, 6%)
7. pH of dissolution medium (0.1 N HCl, Distilled water, Phosphate buffer pH 6.8)
8. Stirring speed of dissolution medium (50 rpm, 100 rpm, 150 rpm)
9. Storage conditions at 25 °C and 40 °C for 3 months

In-vitro Evaluations

For microparticles:
1. Micromeritics
2. Size and shape study (by SEM)
3. Entrapment efficiency
4. Production yield
5. Interaction studies by FTIR, XRD and DSC
6. Dissolution

For tabletted microparticles:
1. Weight variation
2. Thickness variation
3. Friability
4. Hardness
5. Tablet chemical assay
6. Dissolution
7. Swelling and erosion study

In-vivo Evaluation

For tabletted microparticles:

HPLC method development:
1. Optimization of variables
2. Method validation
3. Application of optimized validated

For tabletted microparticles:

Pharmacokinetic and bioavailability study,

IVIVC development

3.1 Materials

Salbutamol sulphate, diclofenac sodium and tramadol hydrochloride were gifted by Unexo Laboratories, Sami Pharmaceuticals and Ali Gohar Pharmaceuticals, Pakistan, respectively. Bamethan sulphate (BS), polyisobutylene (PIB) and ethyl cellulose (EC, 22 cp) were purchased from Sigma (USA). Potassium dihydrogen phosphate (KH_2PO_4), n-hexane, toluene, cyclohexane, acetone, ammonium dihydrogen phosphate ($(NH_4)H_2PO_4$), acetonitrile (CH_3CN), Methanol (CH_3OH), phosphoric acid (H_3PO_4), ammonium acetate (CH_3COONH_4), acetic acid (CH_3COOH), hydrochloric acid (HCl), sodium dihydrogen phosphate (NaH_2PO_4), di(2-ethylhexyl) phosphate (DEHP) and perchloric acid ($HClO_4$) were supplied by Merck (Germany) and tri-ethylamine (TEA) by Fluka (Switzerland). Chloroform, light Mineral oil, petroleum ether (40-60°C) and sodium dodecyl sulphate (SDS) were provided by BDH (UK). Human blood was obtained from healthy human volunteers from Bahawal Victoria Hospital, Bahawalpur, Pakistan. Distilled water was prepared in Instruments laboratory, the Islamia of University Bahawalpur, Pakistan. All other chemicals were purchased through commercial sources and were used without further purification.

3.2 Apparatus

The following instruments were used in the research: Magnetic stirrer (Velp, Europe), Oven (Memmert, Germany), Scanning electron microscope, Electronic balance (Precisa, Switzerland), Digital tablet hardness tester (Curio, Pakistan), Digital tablet thickness tester (Curio, Pakistan), Dissolution apparatus (Pharma test, Germany), Milli pore filters (Pharma test, Germany), Automatic sample collector (Pharma Test, Germany), UV-Visible spectrophotometer (Shimadzu 1601, Japan), FTIR spectroscopy (Shimadzu, Japan), High-Performance Liquid Chromatographic System (Agilent Technologies, 1200 Series, USA), Fluorescent detector (FLD, G1321A,

Agilent Technologies, USA), Hettich centrifuge (Tuttlingen, Germany), pH meter (Inolab, Germany), Lichrosorb RP-C18 stainless steel analytical column (4.6 × 200mm, 5 µm) (Agilent, USA), Cellulose acetate filter (0.45 µm pore size, Sartorius, Goettingen, Germany), Sonicator (Elma, Germany).

3.3 METHODS

3.3.1 Preparation of Tablets by Direct Compression

Salbutamol sulphate tablets were prepared by direct compression technique using different EC concentration. SS, EC and lactose were passed through a sieve (No. 20) and then mixed for 5 min. The powder mixture was mixed and ground using mortar and pestle. Lubricants (magnesium stearate and talc) were added and mixed for 2 min. The final lubricated blend was then compressed into tablets using a single-punch tablet machine (Emmy, Pakistan). The compression force was kept constant for all formulations, to eliminate its effect on dissolution. All three tablet formulations, prepared by direct compression, are mentioned in table 3.1. Each tablet contained 8 mg SS. The quantity of EC was 8 mg, 16 mg and 24 mg in tablet formulations W_1, W_2 and W_3, respectively. Tablet weight was kept at 200 mg.

3.3.2 Preparation of Tablet Formulations by Microencapsulation

3.3.2.1 Preparation of Microcapsules

3.3.2.1.1 Microencapsulation by Coacervation-Thermal Change (CTC)

A weighed amount of EC (22cp, 1g) was dissolved in cyclohexane (20ml) by heating to 80°C with vigorous stirring. In this solution, weighed amount of finely pulverized SS (1g/2g/3g) was dispersed. Vigorous stirring was continued throughout the process. The temperature was then reduced to induce phase separation using an ice bath. The product obtained was washed twice with n-hexane (100ml) at room temperature, air-dried and passed through sieve no. 40 to separate individual microcapsules (Yazan et al. 1995). M_1, M_2 and M_3 microencapsulated formulations were prepared with 1:1, 1:2 and 1:3 SS:EC ratios.

Table 3.1: Tablet formulations prepared by direct compression

Ingredients	Quantity (mg) of each ingredient per tablet		
	W_1	W_2	W_3
Salbutamol sulphate	8	8	8
Ethylcellulose	8	16	24
Lactose	180	171	162
Talc	2	2	2
Magnesium stearate	1	1	1
Total	200	200	200

3.3.2.1.2 Microencapsulation by Solvent Evaporation (SE)

EC (22cp, 1g) was dissolved in acetone (20ml) and SS (1g/2g/3g) was dispersed in this solution with stirring for 20 minutes. The dispersion was poured into light mineral oil (100ml) containing tween 80 (1.3%) and stirred for 5h at 1100 rpm at room temperature to remove acetone completely by evaporation. The light mineral oil was decanted and the collected microcapsules were washed twice with n-hexane (100ml) at room temperature. The microcapsules were separated by filtration and air dried for 12h (Amperiadou and Georgarakis 1995). M_7, M_8 and M_9 microencapsulated formulations were prepared with 1:1, 1:2 and 1:3 SS:EC ratios.

3.3.2.1.3 Microencapsulation by Coacervation-non solvent addition (CNSA)

Weighed EC (EC, 22cp, 1g) was dissolved in toluene containing polyisobutylene (6% w/w) in a closed beaker with magnetic stirring (Velp, Europe) at 500 rpm for 6 h followed by dispersion of SS (1g/2g/3g) in it. After stirring the system for 15 min, phase separation was induced by adding petroleum benzin (non-solvent). The product was transferred to ice bath for the solidification of microparticles. The microparticles were treated with chilled petroleum benzin five times. The stirring was continued throughout the procedure. Eventually, microparticles were washed with n-hexane and dried in air for 2 hours followed by drying in oven (Memmert, Germany) at 50°C for 4 h. M_4, M_5 and M_6 microencapsulated formulations were prepared with 1:1, 1:2 and 1:3 SS:EC ratios. M_{10} & M_{11} microencapsulated formulations were also prepared by this technique using two other viscosity grades of EC (10 cp and 46 cp) with 1:2 SS:EC ratios, respectively.

3.3.2.2 Preparation of Tablets

Each batch of microcapsules (M_{TH1} to M_{DS3}) was blended with 1% Talc, 0.5% Magnesium stearate and lactose (used as filler). Each blended mixture was compressed separately into tablets (T_{TH1} to T_{DS3}, respectively) by direct compression on a single punch tablet machine. Microcapsules containing 9.6 mg salbutamol sulphate equivalent to 8 mg salbutamol, 50 mg tramadol hydrochloride and 50 mg diclofenac sodium were present in each tablet of SS, TH and DS, respectively. Three batches of tablets were prepared for each formulation of the three drugs.

3.3.3 In-vitro Evaluation of Formulations

3.3.3.1 Physical Study of Microcapsules

The size and shape of prepared microparticles was determined by light and scanning electron microscope.

At the end of each microencapsulation process, microcapsules were weighed immediately (M_1) and after drying to a constant weight (M_2) (Sah 1997).

$$\text{Microcapsule solvation } (\%) = (M_1 / M_2) \times 100$$

Bulk density was determined by following formula (Lachman et al. 1986);

$$\text{Bulk Density} = \text{Sample weight} / \text{Sample volume}$$

Tap density was measured by employing the conventional tapping method using 10 ml measuring cylinder and the number of tapings was reduced to 100 as it was sufficient to bring about a plateau condition. Taped density was calculated by following formula;

$$\text{Tapped density} = \text{Weight of microcapsules} / \text{Volume of microcapsules after}$$
$$\text{100 tapings}$$

Compressibility index was calculated by following formula;

$$Ci = \{(\text{Initial volume} - \text{Final volume}) / \text{Initial volume}\} \times 100$$

Hausnner's ratio, another index of flowability of microcapsules, was calculated by following formula;

Hausnner's ratio = Volume before taping / Volume after taping

Angle of repose was measured by passing microcapsules through a funnel on the horizontal surface. The height (h) of heap formed was measured and radius (r) of cone base was also determined. The angle of repose (θ) was calculated by following formula (Shariff et al. 2007);

$$\theta = \tan^{-1} h / r$$

Where r is the radius and h is the height.

3.3.3.2. Physicochemical Characterization of Tabletted Microcapsules

The tabletted microcapsules were evaluated with respect to different physical parameters. The weight variation was determined on 20 tablets using an electronic balance (Precisa, Switzerland) to verify uniformity and conformity of tablets within each formulation (BP, 2004). Tablet hardness was determined for 10 tablets using a digital tablet hardness tester (Curio, Pakistan) to measure the crushing strength of tablets. Friability was determined with 10 tablets in a cambell electronic friabulator for 5 minutes at 25 rpm. The thickness of the tablets was measured using a digital tablet thickness tester (Curio, Pakistan).

For the determination of active pharmaceutical ingredient, 20 tablets were taken from each batch of tabletted microcapsules to evaluate their drug contents. These tablets were weighed and finely ground separately. An adequate amount of this powder was accurately weighed and repeated the same procedure as mentioned earlier in the assay of microcapsules.

3.3.3.3. Assay

An accurately weighed quantity of microcapsules from each batch was dissolved in small amount of methanol (less than 5 ml) to dissolve EC coat. To it, 15 ml of distilled water was added and the solution was heated to evaporate methanol. Then final volume was made to 25 ml with distilled water, filtered to remove insoluble EC and diluted to make volume upto 450 ml with distilled water. This solution was then analyzed spctrophotometrically at λ_{max} (specific for each drug) against its standard solution exposed to the same conditions. λ_{max} of SS and DS is 276 nm and of TH is 271 nm. Three determinations of the microcapsule drug content from the same batch were made (Sajeev et al. 2002).

The drug loading (%) was calculated using the following equation:

$$\text{Drug loading } (\%) = \frac{\text{Amount of drug found in microparticles}}{\text{Amount of drug used for microencapulation}} \times 100$$

The encapsulation efficiency (%) was determined by the following equation:

$$\text{Encapsulation efficiency } (\%) = \frac{\text{Actual drug loading}}{\text{Theoretical drug loading}} \times 100$$

The percentage production yield of the produced microcapsules was calculated for each batch by dividing the weight of microcapsules (M) by the total expected weight of drug and polymer (M_t):

$$\text{Production yield } (\%) = \frac{M}{Mt} \times 100$$

Each determination was performed in triplicate (Hascicek et al. 2003; Soppimath et al. 2001).

3.3.3.4. In vitro Dissolution Studies

The USP XXIV apparatus I (rotating basket, six replicates, pharma test, Germany) method was used for in vitro dissolution studies of all microcapsules. Distilled water was used as dissolution medium. The rate of stirring was 50 rpm. An accurately weighed quantity of microcapsules containing SS equivalent to 8 mg salbutamol, 50 mg DS or 50 mg TH was obtained and placed in 450 ml of dissolution medium maintained at $37 \pm 1^{\circ}C$. 5 ml of the sample was withdrawn and filtered through milli pore filters (Pharma test, Hainberg, Germany) at 0, 30, 60, 90, 120, 150 and 180 minutes with an automatic sample collector (Pharma Test, Germany). The dissolution media were replaced by 5 ml of fresh dissolution medium to maintain a constant volume in the dissolution flask. The samples of SS were analyzed directly at 276 nm and that of DS and TH after suitable dilution at 271 nm using a UV-Visible spectrophotometer (Shimadzu 1601, Japan). While in vitro dissolution study of various tabletted microcapsules was conducted using USP XXIV apparatus II (rotating paddle, six replicates, Pharma test, Germany) and samples were drawn at pre-determined time intervals (0, 0.5, 1, 1.5, 2, 3, 4, 6, 8, 10 and 12 hours) after filtration through milli pore filters followed by UV spectrophotometeric analysis (USP, 2007).

3.3.3.5. Model analysis and Statistics

3.3.3.5.1. Model dependent approaches

The methods investigated to compare drug release profiles can be classified into two categories: model dependent approaches and model independent approaches. Five model-dependent approaches (Zero order, First order, Higuchi, Hixson-Crowell and Korsmeyer-Peppas) were used to compare drug dissolution profiles and interpret drug release kinetics from all formulations with the help of equations 1-5.

Zero Order Model (Khatun et al. 2004): $\quad\quad M_t = M_0 + K_0 t \quad\quad$ (1)

First Order Model (Khatun et al. 2004): $\quad\quad \ln M_t = \ln M_0 + K_1 t \quad$ (2)

Higuchi Model (Higuchi, 1963): $\quad\quad M_t = M_0 + K_H t_{1/2} \quad$ (3)

Hixson-Crowell Model (Hixson & Crowell 1931): $\quad M_0^{\,3} - M_t^{\,3} = K_{HC} t \quad$ (4)

Korsmeyer-Peppas Model (Korsmeyer et al. 1983): $\quad M_t/M_\alpha = K_k t^n \quad$ (5)

In these equations, M_t is the cumulative amount of drug released at any specified time point and M_0 is the initial amount of drug in the formulation. K_0, K_1, K_H, K_{HC} and K_k are rate constants for zero order, first order, Higuchi, Hixson-Crowell and Korsmeyer-Peppas models, respectively. In equation (5), M_t/M_α is the fraction of drug release at time t and n is the release exponent that characterizes different release mechanisms. The n-value is calculated from the slope of Korsmeyer-Peppas plot.

3.3.3.5.2. Model independent approaches

While ANOVA based procedures and pair wise procedures are the model independent approaches which are also exercised in this research work. For this purpose, one way ANOVA plus Post-Hoc analysis (Duncan and Tukey) for significance at $P < 0.05$ was conducted for whole release profiles using SPSS version 12.0 (Polli et al. 1996). Pair wise procedures include the difference factor (f_1) [Eq. (6)] and the similarity factor (f_2) [Eq. (7)]. According to the FDA guidance, values of f_1 between zero and 15 and of f_2 between 50 and 100 ensure sameness or equivalence of the two dissolution profiles. In both equations, R_t and T_t represent the dissolution measurements at P time points of the reference and test, respectively (Koester et al. 2004).

$$f_1 = \left\{ \left[\sum_{i=1}^{P} \left| R_t - T_t \right| \right] / \left[\sum_{i=1}^{P} R_t \right] \right\} \quad\quad (6)$$

$$f_{2=}50 \log \left\{[1+ (1/P)\sum_{i=1}^{P} (R_t-T_t)^2]^{-1/2} *100\right\}$$

(7)

3.3.3.6. UV and FTIR spectroscopy

Drug-polymer interaction was studied by UV spectroscopy. For this purpose, UV spectra of the following solutions were recorded in the range of 200-400 nm using UV-Visible spectrophotometer (Shimadzu 1601, Japan): (i) Pure SS solution in distilled water, (ii) Pure EC solution and (iii) The solution prepared for the determination of drug entrapment efficiency of drug loaded microparticles. SS, EC and microparticles were also evaluated using FTIR spectroscopy (MIDAC M2000, USA) by KBr disc method. FTIR spectrum of each sample was taken in the range of 500-4500 cm^{-1}.

3.3.3.7. Thermal analysis

Thermal analysis [differential scanning calorimetry (DSC), thermogravimetric analysis (TGA) and differential thermometric analysis (DTA)] of microparticles and its individual components was conducted by using TA Instruments (USA). Accurately weighed samples were heated on alumina pan at a constant rate of 10°C/min under a nitrogen flow of 40 ml/min.

3.3.3.8. X-ray diffractometry

X-ray powder diffractometric analysis of microparticles and its individual components was carried out by using D8 Discover (Bruker, Germany) to find out any change in the crystallinity of drug during microencapsulation. The samples were scanned from 8° to 70° diffraction angle range under the following conditions: Cu-K$_\infty$ radiation 1.5406 A° (source), 4°/min scan speed, scintillation detector, primary slit 1 mm, secondary slit 0.6 mm.

3.3.3.9. Estimation of swelling and Erosion of Tabletted Microparticles

SS-EC tabletted microparticles were also evaluated for their swelling and erosion behavior to verify anomalous diffusion (Al-Taani & Tashtoush 2003). Each tablet matrix was weighed before and after dissolution in above mentioned specific conditions for particular time and after drying at 40°C for 48 h to determine their erosion. Swelling (%) and erosion (%) was estimated by following formulas;

Swelling (%) = S/R × 100   (8)

Erosion (%) = (T - R)/T × 100   (9)

Where T is initial weight of the matrix; S is weight of the matrix after swelling; and R is the weight of eroded matrix.

3.3.3.10 Batch Reproducibility and Stability on Storage

Three batches of microcapsules with different drug polymer ratio were prepared and their dissolution rates and drug contents were evaluated under the same conditions as given above. A particular number of microcapsules from each batch were packed in air tight amber glass bottles and stored at 25°C and 40°C. The drug contents and the dissolution behavior of microcapsules were tested monthly for three months following the same procedure as described previously.

3.3.4 In-vivo Evaluation

3.3.4.1 Chromatographic conditions

A Lichrosorb RP-C18 stainless steel analytical column (4.6 × 200mm, 5 µm) (Agilent, USA) was used. HPLC system was operated at room temperature. Mobile phase of following composition CH_3OH:$(NH_4)H_2PO_4$ (67 mM) (pH 3.0 adjusted with

H_3PO_4) : TEA, 50 : 50 : 0.02 (v/v/v%) was prepared, filtered through Cellulose Acetate Filter (0.45 µm pore size, Sartorius, AG37070 Goettingen, Germany) and degassed by sonicator (T490DH, Elma, Germany) at 70 Hz before use. Mobile phase was delivered at a rate of 0.7 mL/min. Injection volume was 100 µl. FLD was operated at excitation wavelength 228 nm and emission wavelength 310 nm.

3.3.4.2 Preparation of samples

100 mg of SS was dissolved in 100 mL of double distilled water to produce its stock solution (1mg/mL). Then it was diluted to 5, 10, 50, 100, 200, 400 and 800 ng/mL (SS working standard solutions) by adding mobile phase. Similarly, 2µg/mL working standard solution of internal standard (TH) was prepared from its stock solution (1mg/mL). Spiked plasma standards (0.5, 1.0, 5, 10, 20, 40 and 80 ng/mL) were prepared by adding 100 µl of SS working standard solutions to 860 µl of drug free human plasma received from a healthy young volunteer. 40 µl (4 ng/40 µl) of TH working solution was also added to each concentration. One blank plasma sample (plasma without drug and internal standard) was analyzed with calibration standards. Another set of spiked plasma standards (1.0, 40 and 80 ng/mL) was prepared without internal standard and stored at -20°C to investigate SS stability over a period of 16 days.

3.3.4.3. Optimization Studies

3.3.4.3.1. Process variables

(1) Compositions of solvent mixtures as mobile phase, as given in Table 3.2,

(2) concentration of $(NH_4)H_2PO_4$ (47; 57; 67 mM),

(3) volume percent of CH_3CN (30; 50; 70),

(4) pH of the mobile phase (3.0; 4.0; 5.0),

(5) excitation and emission wavelengths of FLD,

Table 3.2: Mobile phases and their percentage compositions by volume employed in the development of a HPLC method for the detection of salbutamol sulfate in human plasma

Serial No.	Mobile phases	Compositions (v/v%)
1	$CH_3CN:H_2O$	8:92 and 10:90
2	$CH_3CN:H_2O:H_3PO_4$	8:91.85:0.15
3	$CH_3CN:H_2O:H_3PO_4$	8:91.8:0.2
4	$CH_3CN:H_2O:CH_3OH$	10:70:20
5	$CH_3OH:CH_3COOH:TEA$ (pH 3.0 adjusted with H_3PO_4)	100:0.001:0.001
6	$CH_3CN:NaH_2PO_4$ (40mM)(pH 3.0 adjusted with H_3PO_4)	8:92
7	$CH_3CN:CH_3COONH_4$ (0.1M and 1M)(pH 3.0 adjusted with CH_3COOH)	8:92
8	$CH_3CN:KH_2PO_4$ (40mM)(pH 3.0 adjusted with H_3PO_4)	8:92
9	$CH_3OH:(NH_4)H_2PO_4$ (67mM)(pH 3.0 adjusted with H_3PO_4)	50:50 and 30:70 and 70:30
10	$CH_3OH:(NH_4)H_2PO_4$ (67mM)(pH 3.0 adjusted with H_3PO_4):TEA	50:50:0.02
11	$CH_3CN:(NH_4)H_2PO_4$ (67mM)(pH 3.0 adjusted with H_3PO_4):TEA	50:50:0.02
12	$CH_3OH:(NH_4)H_2PO_4$ (67mM)(pH 3.0 adjusted with H_3PO_4):TEA:SDS	50:50:0.02:0.5
13	$CH_3CN:(NH_4)H_2PO_4$ (67mM)(pH 3.0 adjusted with H_3PO_4):CH_3OH	4.4:92.2:3.4

(6) flow rate of mobile phase (0.5; 0.7; 0.9),

(7) choice of internal standard (BS, TH, DS)

(8) choice of protein extracting agent (CH_3OH, CH_3CN, DEHP and $HClO_4$) and its amount. Each factor was examined at different levels which were chosen as such and/or smaller and/or higher than the nominal level as determined in the preliminary optimization.

3.3.4.3.2. Sample clean up procedures

3.3.4.3.2.1. Protein Extraction by DEHP

5.5 mL of 0.1 M DEHP in chloroform was added to 1.0 mL plasma sample in 10 mL glass tube. The resultant was agitated gently in the upright position on a vortex mixer for 10 min followed by centrifugation at 2000 rpm for 10 min. The chloroform layer was shifted to another 10 mL glass tube already containing 1 mL of 0.5 M HCl. The resultant was agitated gently as before for 10min, and then centrifuged at 2000 rpm for 10 min. A 100 µl aliquot of the acidic layer was injected into the sample loop of HPLC manually. Then unextracted standards were also prepared in 0.5 M HCl to determine extraction efficiency. The clear supernatant layer was then injected to the HPLC system.

3.3.4.3.2.2. Protein Extraction by CH_3OH/ CH_3CN/ $HClO_4$

To 1.0 mL plasma sample in a glass tube, 1 mL of CH_3OH or CH_3CN or 30 µl of $HClO_4$ was added. The resultant was vortexed gently for 10 min and centrifuged at 2000 rpm for 10 min. The protein precipitates down and an aliquot of 100 µl of clear layer were injected into HPLC manually. Their unextracted samples were then prepared to determine extraction efficiency. The clear supernatant layer was then injected to the HPLC system.

3.3.4.4. Validation of the Method

After development and optimization of a chromatographic method, it must be validated in the light of FDA guidelines (FDA, 2000) i.e. specificity, accuracy, precision, linearity (calibration curve), range, detection limit (LOD), quantitation limit (LOQ), robustness, ruggedness, extraction efficiency and stability.

3.3.4.5. Application to study pharmacokinetics

The method narrated above was applied to quantify the plasma concentration of SS in a single dose pharmacokinetic study. Twenty four healthy male adult non-smoker Pakistani human subjects weighing (61-85 kg) and having no clinical and biological abnormality were selected after screening through haemodynamic, haematological and urinalytical evaluation and divided into 4 groups (A, B, C and D), each consisting of 6 subjects (Reports 3.1-3.4). In first sampling, group A, B and C received T_1, T_2 and T_3 formulations respectively and 4th group received reference one (Ventolin 8 mg SR, Glaxosmithkline, Pakistan) with water after a full night fast. The complete sampling schedule is given below:

	Sampling 1	Sampling 2	Sampling 3	Sampling 4
Formulation T_1	Group A	Group D	Group C	Group B
Formulation T_2	Group B	Group A	Group D	Group C
Formulation T_3	Group C	Group B	Group A	Group D
Formulation Reference	Group D	Group C	Group B	Group A

A wash out period of one week was set between each sampling phase. Lunch and dinner was provided after 4 h and 8 h post dosing time, respectively. The ethics of this study were approved by the Board of Advance Studies and Research, the Islamia University of Bahawalpur. After drug administration, 5 mL blood samples were drawn through an indwelling intravenous canula at a predose and at 0, 0.5, 1.0, 1.5,

2.0, 3.0, 4.0, 5.0, 6.0, 8.0, 10.0, 12.0 and 24 h followed by centrifugation immediately at 3500 rpm for 10 minutes. Plasma was separated and stored at $-20°C$ until analysis.

3.3.4.6. Pharmacokinetic analysis

Previously obtained data was tabulated in a Microsoft Excel worksheet, plasma drug concentration-time curve was plotted and different pharmacokinetic parameters i.e. AUC, t_{max} and C_{max} etc, were calculated.

3.3.4.7. Statistical analysis

ANOVA based procedures was also exercised in this research work. For this purpose, one way ANOVA for significance at $P < 0.05$ was conducted for in-vivo data using SPSS version 12.0.

Report 3.1: Biochemical tests of the subjects participated in the in-vivo studies of salbutamol sulphate administered in oral dose of 8 mg tablets SR in Healthy Human Volunteers (Before study)

Urine Examination	Volunteers / Subjects Participated in the Study											
Physical	1	2	3	4	5	6	7	8	9	10	11	12
Volume	22ml	15ml	22ml	32ml	26ml	70ml	80ml	40ml	50ml	40ml	40ml	30ml
Colour	yellow	yellow	Yellow	Yellow	Yellow	yellow	yellow	yellow	yellow	yellow	yellow	yellow
Clarity	Clear	clear	Clear	Clear	Clear	clear	clear	clear	clear	clear	clear	clear
Turbidity	NiL	NiL	NiL	NiL	NiL	NiL	NiL	NiL	NiL	NiL	NiL	NiL
Specific Gravity	1.025	1.004	1.001	1.002	1.001	1.02	1.01	1.03	1.00	1.001	1.001	1.001
Chemical												
PH	Acidic	Acidic	Acidic	Acidic	Acidic	Acidic	Acidic	Acidic	Acidic	Acidic	Acidic	Acidic
Albumin	NiL	NiL	NiL	NiL	NiL	NiL	NiL	NiL	NiL	NiL	NiL	NiL
Sugar	NiL	NiL	NiL	NiL	NiL	NiL	NiL	NiL	NiL	NiL	NiL	NiL
Ketone bodies	NiL	NiL	NiL	NiL	NiL	NiL	NiL	NiL	NiL	NiL	NiL	NiL
Microscopic												
Pus cells	0-1	2 – 3	2 - 3	2 – 3	0-1	0-1	1 – 2	0-1	NiL	0-2	2-4	2 – 3
Red cells	NiL	NiL	NiL	NiL	NiL	NiL	NiL	0-1	NiL	NiL	0-1	NiL
Epithelial cells	NiL	a few	1 - 2%	0-1	1 - 2	1 - 2	0-1	1 - 2	NiL	0-1	3-4	NiL
Yeast cells	NiL	NiL	NiL	NiL	NiL	NiL	NiL	NiL	NiL	NiL	NiL	NiL
Mucus thread	NiL	NiL	NiL	NiL	NiL	NiL	NiL	NiL	NiL	NiL	NiL	NiL
Spermatozoa	NiL	NiL	NiL	NiL	NiL	NiL	NiL	NiL	NiL	NiL	NiL	NiL
Crystals	NiL	NiL	NiL	NiL	NiL	NiL	1 - 2	0-1	NiL	2 - 3	6-8	1 - 2
Casts	NiL	NiL	NiL	NiL	NiL	NiL	NiL	NiL	NiL	NiL	NiL	NiL
Organisms	NiL	NiL	NiL	NiL	NiL	NiL	NiL	NiL	NiL	NiL	NiL	NiL
Amorphous urates	NiL	NiL	NiL	NiL	NiL	NiL	NiL	NiL	NiL	NiL	NiL	NiL

Report 3.2: Biochemical tests of the subjects participated in the in-vivo studies of salbutamol sulphate administered in oral dose of 8 mg tablets SR in Healthy Human Volunteers (Before study)

Heamatology Reports	Volunteers / Subjects Participated in the Study														
Test	1	2	3	4	5	6	7	8	9	10	11	12	Mean	SD	SEM
Haemoglobin (G/dl)	12.1	12.4	11.4	11.8	11.9	11.7	12.8	12.4	12.3	12.2	11.7	12.7	12.117	0.428	0.124
Total RBCs (x 10^{12}/L)	4.6	4.3	4.2	5	5.3	5.6	5.7	5.1	4.8	4.2	4.6	4.2	4.800	0.543	0.157
HCT (%)	33	34	38	36	42	41	43	46	47	42	43	41	40.500	4.421	1.276
MCH (G/dl)	25	28	28	29	32	30	31	30	30	31	32	32	29.833	2.082	0.601
MCHC(Pgm)	30	31	34	32	35	36	37	35	36	32	35	34	33.917	2.193	0.633
Platelet count (x 10^9/L)	186	190	245	213	163	222	163	170	196	244	259	241	207.66	34.45	9.932
WBC count (x 10^9/L)	10.8	8.7	8.1	7.4	5.9	8.1	8.7	6.2	7.6	8.2	9.8	8.6	8.175	1.358	0.392
ESR(mm/1st Hr)	6	8	10	13	6	18	7	10	8	7	21	7	10.083	4.870	1.406
Neutrophil (%)	67	72	66	66	68	58	71	59	69	54	62	70	65.167	5.686	1.642
Lymphocyte (%)	28	26	30	32	30	37	26	38	40	39	33	26	32.083	5.282	1.525
Monocyte (%)	3	1	2	1	11	4	2	2	2	4	3	2	3.083	2.678	0.773
Eosinophils (%)	2	1	2	1	1	1	2	1	1	1	2	3	1.500	0.674	0.195
Serum Electrolytes															
Sodium	145	142	144	140	141	136	132	134	137	132	131	142	138.00	4.973	1.436
Potassium	3.2	4	3.8	3.6	3.5	3.8	3.4	4	3.3	3.4	3.7	4	3.642	0.284	0.082
Blood Glucose															
Sugar random	107	117	98	99	103	102	104	97	98	117	123	102	105.53	8.702	2.512

Report 3.3: Biochemical tests of the subjects participated in the in-vivo studies of salbutamol sulphate administered in oral dose of 8 mg tablets SR in Healthy Human Volunteers (Before study)

Liver Function Test	Volunteers / Subjects Participated in the Study														
Test	1	2	3	4	5	6	7	8	9	10	11	12	Mean	SD	SEM
Bilirubin Total	0.4	0.43	0.6	0.67	0.3	0.95	0.8	0.6	0.8	0.8	1.1	0.4	0.65417	0.24511	0.07071
S.G.P.T	23	22	26	19	27	31	34	24	27	29	39	21	26.833	5.750	1.660
S.G.O.T	35	40	36	38	42	45	30	35	35	40	45	45	38.833	4.840	1.397
Alkaline Phosphatases	192	205	221	178	226	184	219	156	225	168	204	187	197.083	23.306	6.728
Total protein	7.1	6	6.5	6.9	7	6	6.6	6	7	6	7.8	6.5	6.617	0.569	0.164

Renal Function Test

	1	2	3	4	5	6	7	8	9	10	11	12	Mean	SD	SEM
Creatinine	0.5	0.5	0.4	0.3	0.3	0.9	1	0.7	0.7	0.5	1	1.2	0.667	0.299	0.086

Viral Hepatitis Report

	1	2	3	4	5	6	7	8	9	10	11	12	Mean	SD	SEM
HbsAg	0.01	0.02	0.01	0.01	0.01	0.011	0.008	0.011	0.003	0.002	0.005	0.001	0.007	0.004	0.001

Report 3.4: Characteristics of the subjects participated in the in-vivo studies of salbutamol sulphate administered in oral dose of 8 mg tablets SR in Healthy Human Volunteers (Before study)

Subject No.	Age (Years)	Weight (Kg)	Height (Cm)	Temperature (F°)	Heart Rate (per min)	Systolic B.P (mm Hg)	Diastolic B.P (mm Hg)
1	22	50	156	98	90	120	70
2	25	55	167	98.4	74	120	80
3	21	60	157	98	72	110	70
4	24	65	158	99	90	100	80
5	23	60	169	98	86	110	80
6	22	58	164	98	74	120	80
7	21	60	165	99	78	110	70
8	35	65	157	98	76	120	70
9	30	70	170	98	87	120	80
10	31	65	168	98	88	120	80
11	24	68	159	98	89	110	80
12	35	70	174	98.4	90	120	70
Sum	26.083	62.167	162.833	98.233	82.833	115.000	75.833
Mean	5.248	6.118	6.279	0.389	7.322	6.742	5.149
SEM	1.515	1.766	1.813	0.112	2.114	1.946	1.487

The cumulative amount of drug absorbed (%) at time t was calculated by Wagner-Nelson method (Emami, 2006);

Percent Absorbed = {(C$_{(t)}$ / Ke + AUC$_{(0-t)}$ / AUC$_{(0-\infty)}$) × 100 (Equation-10)

Where, C$_t$ is plasma concentration at time t and K$_e$ is elimination rate constant. AUC$_{(0-t)}$ and AUC$_{(0-\infty)}$ represent the area under the curve from time zero to time t and infinity, respectively.

3.3.4.7. Internal prediction error

In vivo properties of a drug can be predicted from its relevant initial in vitro dissolution performance by evaluating predictive mathematical IVIVC model, known as internal predictability. Following approach, based on AUC, is used to evaluate the error in internal predictability (Emami, 2006);

Prediction Error (%) = [(AUC$_{observed}$ − AUC$_{predicted}$)/AUC$_{observed}$]×100 (Equation-11)

Results

&

Discussion

4. RESULTS AND DISCUSSION

4.1. Salbutamol Sulphate-Ethylcellulose Microparticles: Formulation and In-Vitro Evaluation with Emphasis on Mathematical Approaches

The non solvent addition-coacervation technique was applied to prepare SS microparticles. Toluene was used as a solvent for EC, whereas SS is toluene insoluble drug. Petroleum ether was used as a non-solvent to induce coacervation. EC was used as a wall-forming material on account of its safety, stability, hydrophobicity and compact film forming nature among water insoluble polymers (Rowe et al., 2003). Although we used same active ingredient and polymer as by Yazan et al. (1995) but we have used different encapsulation technique from reported one. Previously, coacervation by heat change technique was employed but in the present work, non-solvent addition coacervation technique is applied. Moreover, the former authors characterized microcapsules by dissolution only but solvation, micromeritics, swelling & erosion study, dissolution and drug-polymer interaction study were made in the present study to characterize microcapsules. In addition, the study was concentrated on the effect of SS & EC ratio, PIB, HPMC, dissolution media and stirring speed on formulations.

4.1.1. Physicochemical Characterization of Microparticles

The microparticles were whitish, aggregated and irregular in shape. It is evident from Table 4.1 and Figure 4.1 that there is an increasing ($p > 0.05$) trend in particle size with an increase in EC concentration. This increase in size can be attributed to the increased aggregation of particles with an increase in its

Table 4.1: Evaluation of physical characteristics of salbutamol sulphate microparticles

Formulations	SS : EC Ratio	PIB Concentration (%)	Drug Loading (%)		Size (Mean Diameter) (M ± S.D) μm	Entrapment (%)	Hydration rate (%)	Production yield (M ± S.D)%	t$_{60\%}$ (M ± S.D) (hrs)
			Theoretical	Actual					
M$_1$	1:1	6	50.00	48.49 ± 0.68	68.37 ± 19.31	96.68	158.34	97.48 ± 1.21	0.85
M$_2$	1:2	6	33.33	32.22 ± 1.41	70.04 ± 27.15	96.98	176.09	98.19 ± 1.20	1.44
M$_3$	1:3	6	25.00	24.46 ± 1.29	72.01 ± 19.71	97.83	182.36	98.33 ± 1.37	2.93
M$_4$	1:2	9	33.33	32.33 ± 0.96	69.83 ± 22.64	97.01	172.85	98.14 ± 1.16	1.55
M$_5$	1:2	12	33.33	32.41 ± 1.31	69.68 ± 29.16	97.23	169.34	98.35 ± 1.08	1.72

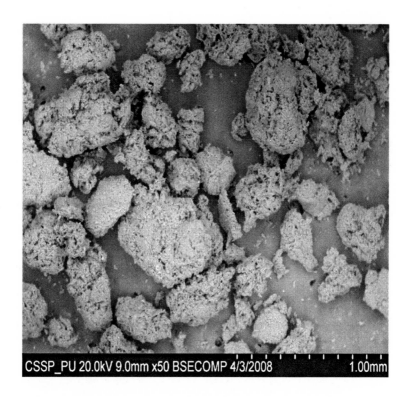

CSSP_PU 20.0kV 9.0mm x50 BSECOMP 4/3/2008   1.00mm

Figure 4.1: Scanning electron micrographs of salbutamol sulpahte-
ethylcellulose microparticles (M_1)

concentration. Same observations were reported by Amperiadou and Georgarakis (1995) and Sajeev et al. (2002). It was analyzed that the encapsulation efficiency is influenced by core to wall ratio. With increasing EC ratio, more particles of SS are coated with it which leads to a higher encapsulation efficiency and certifies previous results (Breghausen et al., 2002; Singh and Robinson, 1990). However, this increase is not significant statistically (p>0.05). An increase in EC concentration caused a slight increase in production yield of microparticles (p>0.05). A little increase in encapsulation efficiency and production yield and slight decrease in particle size is observed by increase in PIB contents from 6-12% during microencapsulation process (p>0.05) as mentioned previously (Yazan et al., 2002; Amperiadou and Georgarakis, 1995).

Rheological properties of all formulations are expressed in terms of bulk density, taped density, compressibility index, Hausner's ratio and angle of repose (Table 4.2). It was observed that bulk density decreased with an increase in drug polymer ratio. Present results are in agreement with that reported by Shariff et al. (2007) who has also reported that bulk density increased when the polymer concentration was decreased. Compressibility index of all six formulations is below 15% indicating excellent flow properties. Hausner's ratio for all formulations was below 1.29 indicating free flow of all formulations of microcapsules and similarly angle of repose for all formulations are below 30° indicating once again free flowing nature of microcapsules.

Table 4.2: Rheological properties of microcapsules

Formulations	Bulk density (g/ml)	Taped density (g/ml)	Compressibility index (%)	Hausner's ratio	Angle of repose
M_1	0.21	0.23	11.00	1.16	21.87°
M_2	0.26	0.31	12.87	1.09	23.94°
M_3	0.30	0.33	10.39	1.29	27.45°
M_4	0.29	0.29	13.15	1.03	28.68°
M_5	0.24	0.26	13.62	1.17	25.13°

4.1.2. Physical Characterization of Tablets

Physical attributes of the tablets i.e. physical appearance, tablet hardness, weight variation, tablet thickness, friability and drug content uniformity of the tabletted microcapsules were found to be satisfactory as shown in Table 4.3. Tablet hardness varied between 8.3 ± 1.2 to 9.5 ± 1.1 kg/cm^2 and friability was less than 0.5% (w/w). The designed tablets showed low weight variation (< $\pm$ 3.0%). The average thickness was 3.87 to 3.89 mm. The results fulfilled the requirements of BP 2004.

4.1.3. In Vitro Dissolution Studies

4.1.3.1. Model independent approaches

Salbutamol sulphates tablets were prepared by two methods: (i) by direct compression (W_2) and (ii) by compressing microparticles (M_2). W_2, M_2 and reference tablets (Ventolin 8 mg SR) were tested by dissolution. Very rapid release of drug was observed from W_2 as compared to other two tablets i.e. though each tablet contained 8 mg salbutamol sulphate. More than 90% drug release from W_2 occurred within 6 hours (Figure 4.2). This result showed the need to develop SS sustained-release formulation to achieve prolonged effect. The tabletted microparticles were also evaluated by different mathematical kinetic models, the difference & similarity factors and one way ANOVA plus Post-Hoc Tests. Comparison between dissolution profiles of SS microparticles showed that 60% release of SS was achieved after 0.85, 1.44 and 2.93 hours when drug polymer ratio was 1:1, 1:2 and 1:3, respectively.

Table 4.3: Evaluation of physical properties of salbutamol sulphate tablets

Formulations	Drug Contents (mg)	HPMC Concentration (%)	Weight Variation [a] (%) (± S.D) (n=20)	Thickness (mm) (M ± S.D) (n=10)	Hardness (Kg/cm^2) (M ± S.D) (n=10)	Friability (%) (n=10)	$t_{60\%}$ (hrs)
W_1	9.6[•]	0	± 2.3	3.89 ± 0.04	9.1 ± 1.4	0.32 ± 0.2	1.47
W_2	9.6[•]	0	± 2.8	3.87 ± 0.02	9.4 ± 0.9	0.41 ± 0.5	1.91
W_3	9.6[•]	0	± 2.1	3.88 ± 0.05	8.9 ± 0.06	0.37 ± 0.3	2.39
T_1	9.6[•]	0	± 2.8	3.88 ± 0.04	9.2 ± 1.3	0.36 ± 0.2	4.78
T_2	9.6[•]	0	± 2.7	3.89 ± 0.03	8.5 ± 0.9	0.43 ± 0.2	6.93
T_3	9.6[•]	0	± 2.1	3.88 ± 0.02	8.3 ± 1.2	0.29 ± 0.3	11.05
T_4	9.6[•]	3	± 2.2	3.87 ± 0.08	9.3 ± 1.5	0.39 ± 0.2	8.13
T_5	9.6[•]	6	± 2.1	3.89 ± 0.04	9.5 ± 1.1	0.44 ± 0.4	11.93
Reference Tablet	9.6[•]	Unknown	± 1.4	3.87 ± 0.02	8.7 ± 0.7	0.31 ± 0.1	7.57

[a] ± Maximum% variation from the arithmetic mean

[•] Equivalent to 8 mg Salbutamol

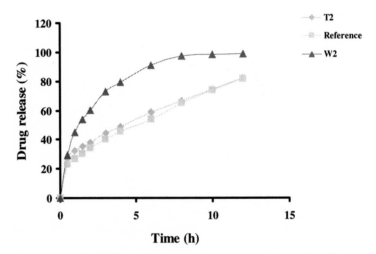

Figure 4.2: The dissolution profiles of salbutamol sulphate tablets (W_2, reference and T_2)

According to Duncan test, $t_{60\%}$ of all batches of the microparticles lied in the same homogenous group (1:1=1:2=1:3) ($p>0.05$) whereas Tukey H.S.D. similarized the $t_{60\%}$ of 1:1 and 1:2 and differentiated them from that of 1:3 but not significantly ($p>0.05$). According to difference factor (f_1) and similarity factor (f_2), the release profiles of following pairs of microparticle formulations are different from each other: M_1 VS M_3 and M_2 VS M_3 as their $f_1>15.00$ and $f_2<50.00$. While M_1 VS M_2 has $f_1<15.00$ and $f_2>50.00$ that indicates the mutual similarity of the compared release profiles but to a very less extent. The results indicated that velocity of drug release was slower from microparticles with low polymer concentration i.e. microparticles having low core to wall ratio and vice versa. It can, therefore, be assumed that decrease in core to wall ratio increased the wall thickness of microparticles and/or decreased the number of surface pores as evident from Figure 4.3. As mentioned earlier, microparticles with low polymer concentration were smaller in size which provided a larger surface area for faster drug release. This result is in accordance with modified Noyes-Whitney equation (Bakan et al., 1986):

$$(dc/dt) = kS \ (Cs - Ct)$$

Where dc/dt is the rate of dissolution, k is the dissolution rate constant, S is the surface area of dissolving body and Cs – Ct is the concentration gradient. Above mentioned results also revealed that the nature of drug changed from crystalline to amorphous during microencapsulation. Since, the amorphous form of a drug is usually more soluble than the crystalline form. Therefore, the release of drug from microparticles is quicker than other dosage forms that satisfy immediate therapeutic effect. Moreover, it is reported previously that release of hydrophilic drugs is mainly controlled by permeation through water filled channels within the hydrophobic polymer membrane. Both of the above mentioned reasons can cause a

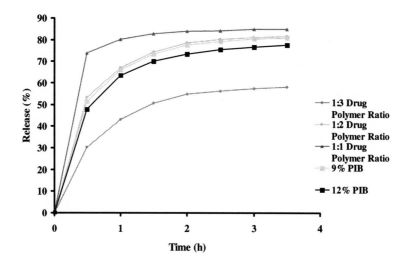

Figure 4.3: The dissolution profiles of salbutamol sulphate microparticles in distilled water showing the effect of drug polymer ratio and the concentration of PIB used in microencapsulation, on dissolution fashion.

deceleration in the diffusion of dissolution medium through these channels that consequently decrease the rate of drug release from microparticles and subsequently from tabletted microparticles (Amperiadou and Georgarakis, 1995; Barik et al., 2001; Breghausen et al., 2002) ($p<0.05$). The corresponding data is presented in Table 4.4. Although there is slight difference among different formulations with respect to their entrapment efficiency but there is comparatively greater variation on the basis of their release kinetics. In this course, M_2 is the best formulation with optimum entrapment efficiency and release profile.

The observed in-vitro drug release profiles from SS microparticles were biphasic: an initial rapid drug release phase (burst) was followed by the slow and prolonged phase. The burst effect may be beneficial because a high initial release produces an instant effect which can be subsequently maintained for a prolonged period by a slower but continuous release of drug.

The rank order of drug/polymer ratios for percentage drug burst was in the order of: 1:1>1:2>1:3, as visible from Figure 4.3 & 4.4. The rapid initial phase of release was thought to occur mainly by dissolution and diffusion of drug entrapped close to or at the surface of microparticles. The second and slower release phase was thought to involve the diffusion of drug entrapped within the inner part of polymer matrix by means of aqueous channels of a network of pores. It has already been reported that an initial burst effect in release profile was observed especially (a) when the drug solubility is high, (b) loading dose in the polymeric matrix is large and (c) lack of critical polymer concentration.

Table 4.4: Release rate parameters [Y-equation (Y=aX + b), determination co-efficient (R^2), correlation co-efficient (r) and release exponent (n)] for release data after fitting of the whole release profiles of salbutamol sulphate from its microparticles into different mathematical models.

Models	Formulations	M_1	M_2	M_3	M_4	M_5
Zero Order	Y-equation	15.723x + 44.274	17.965x + 33.09	13.977x + 19.367	17.98x + 32.107	17.278x + 30.322
	R^2	0.434	0.627	0.728	0.639	0.645
	r	0.659	0.792	0.853	0.799	0.803
First Order	Y-equation	0.760x + 2.5255	0.7979x + 2.3583	0.7747x + 2.0498	0.7999x + 2.3407	0.7945x + 2.3069
	R^2	0.357	0.411	0.464	0.416	0.420
	r	0.597	0.641	0.681	0.645	0.648
Higuchi	Y-equation	5.1976x + 23.829	5.4628x + 14.121	13.977x + 19.367	42.146x + 13.366	40.395x + 12.438
	R^2	0.717	0.877	0.728	0.885	0.889
	r	0.847	0.936	0.853	0.941	0.943
Hixson-Crowell	Y-equation	-0.4332x + 3.6203	-0.4858x + 3.9978	-0.2952x + 4.3068	0.8121x + 2.2215	0.8025x + 2.1792
	R^2	0.518	0.749	0.786	0.448	0.451
	r	0.720	0.865	0.887	0.669	0.672
Korsmeyer-peppa	Y-equation	0.7259x + 3.5222	0.8469x + 3.3658	0.8933x + 2.9953	0.8564x + 3.3473	0.8568x + 3.3039
	R^2	0.095	0.135	0.179	0.139	0.142
	r	0.308	0.367	0.423	0.373	0.377
	n	0.73	0.85	0.89	0.86	0.86

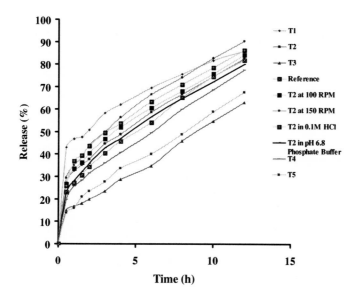

Figure 4.4: The dissolution profiles of salbutamol sulphate tabletted microparticles   showing the effect of HPMC, stirring speed and type of dissolution media on dissolution fashion.

Additionally, when polymer concentration is low, the hydrated polymeric matrix would be highly porous leading to rapid diffusion of the drug from polymeric matrix (Erden and Celebi, 1996; Singh and Robinson, 1990).

4.1.3.2. Model dependent approaches

To get meaningful information, the whole drug release profiles were evaluated kinetically and the best fit of release profiles to zero order, first order, Higuchi, Hixson-Crowell and Korsmeyer-Peppas models was investigated (Table 4.4 & 4.5, Figure 4.3 & 4.4). Model with the highest co-efficient of determination (R^2) was judged to be a more appropriate model for the dissolution data. The release profiles from all the formulations were best explained by Higuchi model due to the highest linearity, followed by zero order and first order, respectively. This finding is in agreement with the previously published results (Yazan et al., 1995; Amperiadou and Georgarakis, 1995). It suggests that drug release is controlled by the diffusion of drug through pores and not through swollen EC.

From Korsmeyer-Peppas model, it is found that the mode of release from all microparticles and tabletted microparticles was anomalous diffusion (non-Fickian, a combination of the diffusion and erosion mechanism). The application of release profiles to the Hixson-Crowell equation indicated a change in surface area and diameter of the formulation with progressive dissolution of matrix as a function of time.

Table 4.5: Release rate parameters [Y-equation (Y=aX + b), determination co-efficient (R^2), correlation co-efficient (r) and release exponent (n)] for release data after fitting of the whole release profiles of salbutamol sulphate from its tabletted microparticles into different mathematical models.

Models	Formulations	T_1	T_2	T_3	T_4	T_5	Reference
Zero Order	Y-equation	5.0685x + 35.772	5.468x + 22.117	4.418x + 11.164	5.3638x + 16.371	4.9022x + 10.526	5.6992x + 18.46
	R^2	0.709	0.883	0.954	0.932	0.963	0.923
	R	0.842	0.940	0.977	0.965	0.981	0.961
First Order	Y-equation	0.1615x + 3.0436	0.182x + 2.712	4.418x + 11.164	0.1911x + 2.5195	0.2028x + 2.2336	0.1909x + 2.6022
	R^2	0.271	0.372	0.484	0.430	0.515	0.414
	R	0.521	0.986	0.696	0.656	0.718	0.643
Higuchi	Y-equation	2.795x + 18.56	2.8179x + 6.3263	2.1794x - 0.2247	20.872x + 1.8611	18.722x - 2.0925	2.8812x + 2.7876
	R^2	0.907	0.986	0.975	0.988	0.984	0.991
	R	0.952	0.993	0.987	0.994	0.992	0.995
Hixson-Crowell	Y-equation	-0.1517x + 4.0255	-0.143x + 4.3204	-0.0937x + 4.4887	0.2009x + 2.2636	0.2049x + 2.0003	0.2038x + 2.3455
	R^2	0.976	0.994	0.992	0.508	0.577	0.497
	R	0.988	0.997	0.996	0.713	0.760	0.705
Korsmeyer-peppa	Y-equation	0.6137x + 3.1039	0.6914x + 2.7802	0.7139x + 2.3484	0.7248x + 2.5923	0.7775x + 2.3022	0.7238x + 2.6755
	R^2	0.261	0.358	0.451	0.412	0.505	0.397
	R	0.511	0.598	0.672	0.642	0.711	0.630
	N	0.61	0.69	0.71	0.72	0.77	0.72

4.1.4. Batch Reproducibility and Stability on Storage

No significant difference was observed in the release profiles of different batches of tabletted microparticles, indicating that the manufacturing process used was reliable and reproducible (p>0.05, f_1=0.29, f_2=99.71). Also, the release kinetics remained unaltered for up to three months of storage, and there were no changes in the tablet characteristics suggesting that SS is stable in tabletted microparticles for the above mentioned period. However, it is needed that the stability for a longer period should be conducted.

4.1.5. Influence of Process Variables

Statistical analysis shows that PIB concentration does not affect drug release behavior significantly (p>0.05, f_1<15.00 and f_2>50.00). However, Figure 4.3 shows a slight increase in sustaining effect on drug release from microparticles which can be attributed to the increased formation of numerous tiny discrete coated particles (Barik et al. 2001, SA et al. 1996). The use of HPMC as an excepient during tablet manufacturing process has imposed a retardant effect on the drug release rate from tabletted microparticles due to its binding effect (p<0.05, f_1>15.00 and f_2<50.00). Almost similar pattern of SS release from tabletted microparticles is observed when dissolution medium was either distilled water or 0.1M HCl solution. Whereas a slight decrease in the rate of dissolution is observed when pH 6.8 phosphate buffer was used as dissolution medium (p<0.05, f_1<15.00 and f_2>50.00). The in vitro dissolution is affected insignificantly (p>0.05, f_1<15.00 and f_2>50.00) by stirring speed.

4.1.6. UV and FTIR Spectroscopy

The UV spectra of pure drug solution and the solution prepared for determination of drug entrapment efficiency of drug loaded microparticles were of the same kind. The λ_{max} of pure SS was observed at 276nm on UV spectra of the solution prepared for determination of drug entrapment efficiency of SS loaded microparticles. Some characteristic and prominent peaks of SS were observed in FTIR spectrum. The spectrum of microparticles showed amino, hydroxyl and aromatic stretchings at the same values as in that of pure SS which confirmed drug. No significant alteration in the nature of peaks denied any strong SS-EC interaction when SS was encapsulated into EC coats. The relevant FTIR spectras are given in Figure 4.5.

4.1.7. Thermal Analysis

Thermal analysis showed good stability of SS in the form of microparticles (Figure 4.6). The characteristic, well-recognizable thermal profile of the drug in a specific temperature range was observed. The same thermal behavior was observed in case of its microparticles but with loss of its sharp appearance that indicated a significant reduction of drug crystallinity in the polymer matrix. It indicated the absence of any strong chemical interaction between drug and polymer.

4.1.8. X-ray Diffractometry

X-ray diffractometry revealed amorphous and crystalline nature of pure EC and SS, respectively as shown in diffractograms (Figure 4.7). However, a decrease

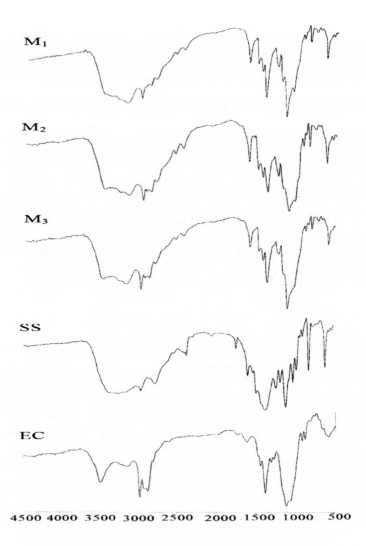

Figure 4.5: FTIR spectras of M_1, M_2 and M_3, salbutamol sulphate and ethylcellulose

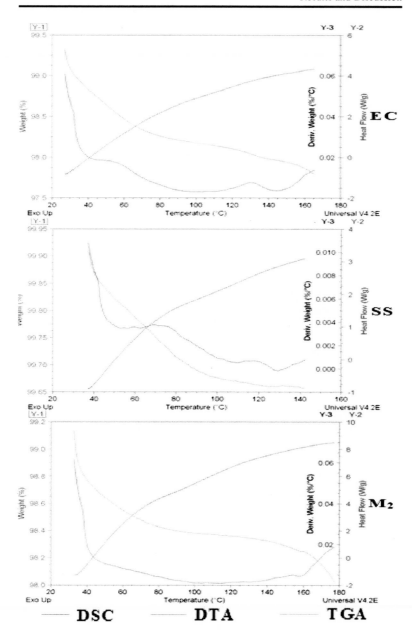

Figure 4.6: Thermal analysis of salbutamol sulphate, ethylcellulose, and formulation M_2

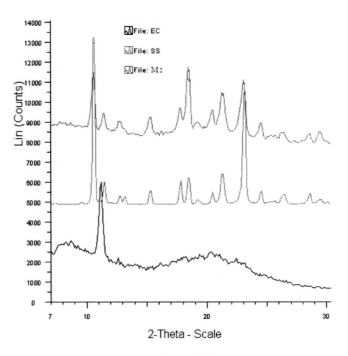

Figure 4.7: X-ray powder diffraction profiles of salbutamol sulphate, ethylcellulose and formulation M_2

in the signal intensity i.e. crystallinity of SS was observed in microparticle form as compared to pure components.

4.1.9. Estimation of Swelling and Erosion of Tabletted Microparticles

The T_2 undergoes swelling and erosion continuously with time (h) after putting into dissolution apparatus as clear from Figure 4.8. This phenomenon is responsible for the gradual release of drug from tabletted microcapsule matrix. It also confirms anomalous diffusion of SS from tabletted microparticles.

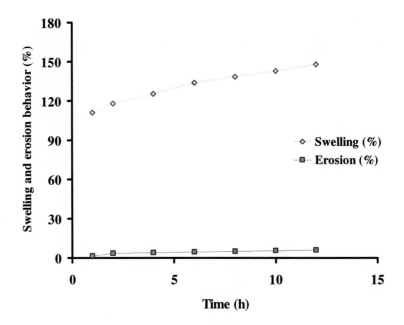

Figure 4.8: Percent erosion and swelling character of T_2. Each data point is a mean ± S.D. of three values.

4.2. Microencapsulation of Tramadol hydrochloride and Physicochemical Evaluation of Formulations

4.2.1. Physicochemical Evaluation of Microparticles

The results of scanning electron microscope showed that microparticles were off white, aggregated and irregular in shape (Figure 4.9). It was found that size (Sajeev et al., 2002; Singh and Robinson, 1990), encapsulation efficiency (Breghausen et al., 2002; Amperiadou and Georgarakis, 1996) and production yield of microparticles increased insignificantly (p>0.5) with an increase in ethocel concentration. However, increase in ethocel concentration produced thick coating around higher number of TH microparticles. It certifies previous findings of Erden & Celebi, (1996) and SA et al., (1996). A little increase in encapsulation efficiency and production yield and slight decrease in particle size (Table 4.6) is observed by increase in PIB contents from 6-12% during microencapsulation process (p>0.05) as mentioned previously (Barik et al., 2001; SA et al., 1996).

Degree of microparticle solvation is affected by solubility properties of solvent (petroleum benzin and n-hexane) and polymer in toluene. During microencapsulation, n-hexane penetrates into matrix due to its solubility in toluene and petroleum benzin. Therefore, resultant microparticles are solvated at the end of process and are less prone to aggregation on drying. Moreover, residual n-hexane should be removed as it can affect adversely the rheological properties. Rheological properties of all formulations are expressed in terms of bulk density, taped density, compressibility index, Hausner's ratio and angle of repose.

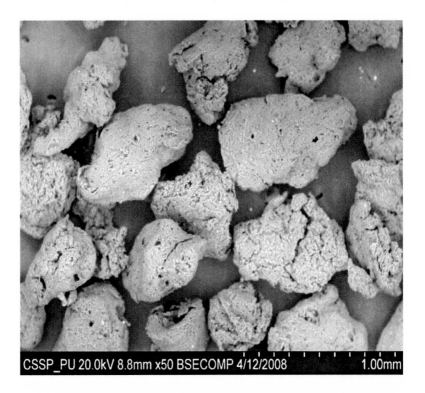

CSSP_PU 20.0kV 8.8mm x50 BSECOMP 4/12/2008   1.00mm

Figure 4.9: Scanning electron micrographs of tramadol hydrochloride microparticles
M_2

Table 4.6: Physicochemical characteristics of tramadol hydrochloride microparticles

Formulations	TH: Ethocel Ratio	PIB Concentration (%)	Entrapment (%)	Production yield (M ± S.D)%	$t_{60\%}$ (M ± S.D) (hrs)	Size (Mean Diameter) (M ± S.D) μm	Solvation rate (%)
M_1	1:1	6	95.43	96.23 ± 1.56	0.86	592.55 ± 19.31	154.75
M_2	1:2	6	96.25	97.20 ± 1.86	1.13	673.95 ± 27.15	164.74
M_3	1:3	6	98.76	97.99 ± 1.24	1.52	722.74 ± 19.71	175.23
M_4	1:2	9	97.21	97.01 ± 1.76	1.42	662.46 ± 22.64	167.64
M_5	1:2	12	96.89	97.64 ± 1.21	1.69	639.56 ± 29.16	159.52

It was observed that bulk density decreased with increase in drug polymer ratio (Table 4.7). Present results are in agreement with previous observation of Shariff et al., (2007) where they have also reported that bulk density increased when the polymer concentration was decreased. Compressibility index of all six formulations is below 15% indicating excellent flow properties. Hausner's ratio and angle of repose were below 1.29 and 30°, respectively for all formulated microparticles again indicating their free flow nature (Sajeev et al., 2002).

4.2.2. Physical Evaluation of Tablets

Physical parameters of the tablets i.e. physical appearance, tablet hardness, weight variation, tablet thickness, friability and drug content uniformity of tabletted microcapsules were found to be satisfactory as shown in Table 4.8. Tablet hardness varied between 8.8 ± 1.2 to 9.4 ± 0.8 kg/cm^2 and friability was less than 0.5% (w/w). The tablets showed low weight variation ($< \pm 3.0\%$). The average thickness was 5.45 mm. The results fulfilled the requirements of B.P. (2004).

4.2.3. In vitro Dissolution Studies

4.2.3.1. Model independent approaches

The microparticles and tablets were evaluated for their release profile in double distilled water. They were also assessed by different mathematical kinetic models, the difference & similarity factors and one way ANOVA plus Post-Hoc Tests. Table 4.6 shows that time for 60% release of TH from M_1, M_2 and M_3 was achieved in 0.86, 1.13 and 1.52 hours, respectively.

Table 4.7: Rheological properties of tramadol hydrochloride microparticles

Formulations	Bulk density (g/ml)	Taped density (g/ml)	Compressibility index (%)	Hausner's ratio	Angle of repose ($\theta°$)
M_1	0.21	0.23	11.0	1.16	21.87
M_2	0.26	0.31	12.87	1.09	23.94
M_3	0.30	0.33	10.39	1.29	27.45
M_4	0.29	0.29	13.15	1.03	28.68
M_5	0.24	0.26	13.62	1.17	25.13

Table 4.8: Physicochemical characteristics of tramadol hydrochloride tablets

Formulations	Drug Contents (mg)	Weight Variation [a] (%) (± S.D) (n=20)	Thickness (mm) (M ± S.D) (n=10)	Hardness (Kg/cm^2) (M ± S.D) (n=10)	Friability (%) (n=10)	t $_{60\%}$ (h)
T$_1$	100	± 2.1	5.46 ± 0.04	9.4 ± 0.8	0.42 ± 0.4	3.47
T$_2$	100	± 2.4	5.44 ± 0.05	8.9 ± 1.1	0.39 ± 0.7	6.26
T$_3$	100	± 2.0	5.47 ± 0.07	9.3 ± 1.4	0.28 ± 0.3	8.90
Reference	100	± 1.9	5.40 ± 0.03	8.3 ± 0.8	0.27 ± 0.2	6.87

[a] Maximum% variation from the arithmetic mean

According to Duncan test, the $t_{60\%}$ of all batches of TH microparticles lied in the same homogenous group ($M_1=M_2=M_3$) while Tukey H.S.D. test similarized the $t_{60\%}$ of M_1 & M_2 and differentiated them insignificantly ($p > 0.05$) from that of M_3. According to difference factor (f_1) and similarity factor (f_2), the release profiles of following pairs of microparticle formulations are different from each other: M_1 VS M_3 and M_2 VS M_3 as their $f_1>15.00$ and $f_2<50.00$. While M_1 VS M_2 has $f_1<15.00$ and $f_2>50.00$ that indicates the mutual similarity of compared release profiles but to a very less extent. The results indicated that rate of drug release was slower from microparticles with low polymer amount i.e. microparticles having low core to wall ratio. It can, therefore, be assumed that decrease in core to wall ratio increased the wall thickness of microparticles and/or decreased the number of surface pores as evident from Figure 4.10. Moreover, it is reported previously that the release of hydrophilic drugs is mainly controlled by permeation through water filled channels within the hydrophobic polymer (Ethocel) membrane. Both of these reasons retard the diffusion of dissolution medium through these channels that ultimately decrease the rate of drug release (Barik et al., 2001; Amperiadou and Georgarakis, 1995; Breghausen et al., 2002).

A biphasic pattern of drug release from TH formulations was observed involving an initial rapid drug release phase (burst) followed by the slow and prolonged phase. Thus, a subsequent prolonged and continuous release of drug can be maintained after an initial high release.

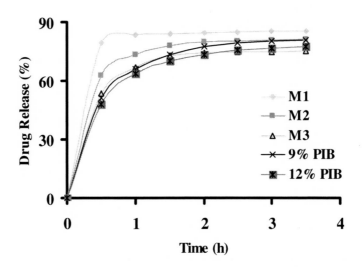

Figure 4.10: The dissolution profiles of tramadol hydrochloride microparticles in distilled water showing the effect of drug polymer ratio and the concentration of PIB used in microencapsulation, on dissolution fashion. Each data point is a mean of three values.

Diffusion of drug bound in the surface region of microparticles was thought to be responsible for burst effect during dissolution, while slow and continuous release was due to the diffusion of drug from core region through a network of channels. Formulation with lowest ethocel concentration showed highest burst effect as evident from Figure 4.10. When polymer concentration is low, the hydrated polymeric matrix would be highly porous leading to rapid diffusion of the drug from polymeric matrix. It has also been reported previously that highly soluble drugs exhibit burst phenomenon more frequently (Singh and Robinson, 1990; Erden and Celebi, 1996).

4.2.3.2. Process variables

Polyisobutylene concentration affected microparticle dissolution profiles insignificantly ($p>0.05$, $f_1<15.00$, $f_2>50.00$) (Figure 4.11) i.e. a slightly slow release profile was observed when PIB concentration was increased. It can be attributed to the increased formation of numerous tiny discrete coated particles (SA et al., 1996; Barik et al., 2001). TH tablet release profiles did not vary when dissolution medium was changed with 0.1M HCl solution. Whereas a slight decrease in the rate of dissolution is observed when pH 6.8 phosphate buffer was used as dissolution medium ($p>0.05$, $f_1<15.00$ and $f_2>50.00$). The stirring speed also affected in vitro dissolution rate insignificantly ($p>0.05$, $f_1<15.00$ and $f_2>50.00$).

4.2.3.3. Model dependent approaches

In order to find best fit kinetic model to the release profiles, dissolution data

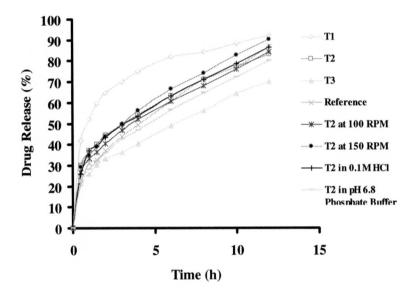

Figure 4.11: The dissolution profiles of tramadol hydrochloride formulated and reference tablets showing the effect stirring speed and type of dissolution media on dissolution fashion. Each data point is a mean of three values.

was characterized kinetically. On the basis of determination co-efficient (R^2), all release profiles found to be best fit to Higuchi model due to highest linearity, followed by zero order and first order, respectively (Table 4.9 and 4.10). It suggests that the drug release is controlled by diffusion of drug through pores and not through the swollen ethocel. The value of "n" further, verified that mechanism of TH release from all formulations was anomalous diffusion i.e. diffusion along with erosion. Hixson-Crowell model showed a change in surface area and diameter of the formulation with progressive dissolution of matrix as a function of time.

4.2.4. Estimation of swelling and Erosion of Tablets

The optimum formulation undergoes swelling and erosion continuously with time (h) in dissolution apparatus as clear from Figure 4.12. This phenomenon is responsible for the gradual release of drug from tablet matrix. It also confirms anomalous diffusion of TH from tabletted microparticles.

4.2.5. Batch Reproducibility and Stability on Storage

No significant ($p > 0.05$, $f_1 = 0.29$, $f_2 = 99.71$) difference was observed in the release pattern of different batches of TH tablets, indicating that the manufacturing process used was reliable and reproducible. Also, the release kinetics remained unaltered for up to three months of storage, and there were no changes in the tablet properties indicating that TH is stable in tabletted microparticles for the above mentioned period.

4.2.6. UV and FTIR Spectroscopy

The UV spectra of pure drug solution and the solution prepared for the

Table 4.9: Release rate parameters [Y-equation (Y=aX + b), determination co-efficient (R^2) and release exponent (n)] for release data after fitting of the whole release profiles of tramadol hydrochloride microparticles into different mathematical models.

Models	Formulations	M_1	M_2	M_3	M_4	M_5
Zero Order	Y-equation	15.03x + 47.07	16.241x + 38.564	15.65x + 34.185	17.98x + 32.107	17.278x + 30.322
	R^2	0.384	0.513	0.546	0.639	0.645
First Order	Y-equation	0.7509x + 2.5612	0.7702x + 2.4447	0.768x + 2.3725	0.7999x + 2.3407	0.7945x + 2.3069
	R^2	0.345	0.378	0.390	0.416	0.420
Higuchi	Y-equation	5.0925x + 26.382	5.1808x + 19.18	4.9241x + 16.135	42.146x + 13.366	40.395x + 12.438
	R^2	0.666	0.790	0.818	0.885	0.889
Hixson-Crowell	Y-equation	-0.4061x + 3.499	-0.4322x + 3.8242	-0.3873x + 3.95	0.8121x + 2.2215	0.8025x + 2.1792
	R^2	0.435	0.613	0.626	0.448	0.451
Korsmeyer-peppa	Y-equation	0.697x + 3.5552	0.7708x + 3.4387	0.7922x + 3.3529	0.8564x + 3.3473	0.8568x + 3.3039
	R^2	0.086	0.110	0.121	0.139	0.142
	N	0.70	0.77	0.79	0.86	0.86

Table-4.10: Release rate parameters [Y-equation (Y=aX + b), determination co-efficient (R^2) and release exponent (n)] for release data after fitting of the whole release profiles of tramadol hydrochloride from its tablets into different mathematical models.

Models	Formulations	T_1	T_2	T_3	Reference
Zero Order	Y-equation	5.1338x + 42.175	5.2952x +26.849	4.6454x + 18.648	5.6992x + 18.46
	R^2	0.627	0.826	0.887	0.923
First Order	Y-equation	0.1584x + 3.1597	0.1733x + 2.8401	0.1773x + 2.582	0.1909x + 2.6022
	R^2	0.248	0.329	0.383	0.414
Higuchi	Y-equation	2.9257x + 23.408	2.7963x + 10.609	2.3851x + 5.3577	2.8812x + 2.7876
	R^2	0.865	0.968	0.983	0.991
Hixson-Crowell	Y-equation	-0.1729x + 3.8694	-0.1434x + 4.2211	-0.107x + 4.3589	0.2038x + 2.3455
	R^2	0.935	0.991	0.998	0.497
Korsmeyer-peppa	Y-equation	0.6116x + 3.209	0.6587x + 2.9049	0.6691x + 2.653	0.7238x + 2.6755
	R^2	0.247	0.317	.364	0.397
	N	0.61	0.66	0.67	0.72

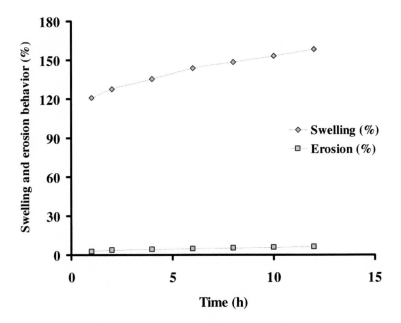

Figure 4.12: Percent erosion and swelling character of optimum formulation T_2. Each data point is a mean of three values.

determination of drug entrapment efficiency of drug loaded microparticles were of the same kind. The λ_{max} of TH, in pure and encapsulated form, was observed at 271 nm. Common characteristic and prominent peaks of TH, in pure and encapsulated form, were observed in FTIR spectrum (Figure 4.13) that denied any strong TH-ethocel interaction when TH was encapsulated into ethocel coats.

4.2.7. X-Ray Diffractometry

X-Ray patterns of pure TH and TH loaded microparticles showed that intensity of pure TH was sharp but when TH was incorporated in microparticles, sharpness of its peaks slightly decreased indicating insignificant change in crystalline structure of TH (Figure 4.14).

4.2.8. Thermal Analysis

Thermal analysis showed good stability of TH in the form of microparticles (Figure 4.15). The characteristic, well-recognizable thermal profile of the drug in a specific temperature range was observed. The same thermal behavior was observed in case of its microparticles but with loss of its sharp appearance that indicated a significant reduction of drug crystallinity in the polymer matrix. It indicated the absence of any strong chemical interaction between drug and polymer.

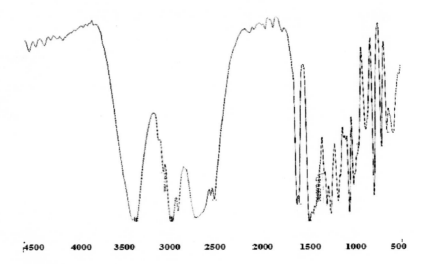

Figure 4.13: FTIR spectra of tramadol hydrochloride formulation (M$_2$)

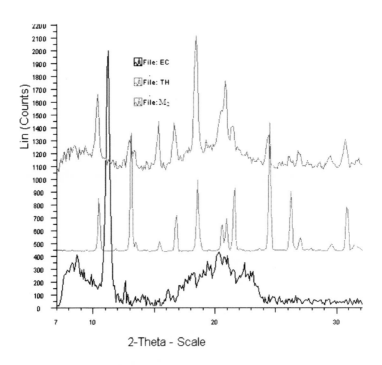

Figure 4.14: X-ray diffractometric spectras of tramadol hydrochloride, ethylcellulose and M_2

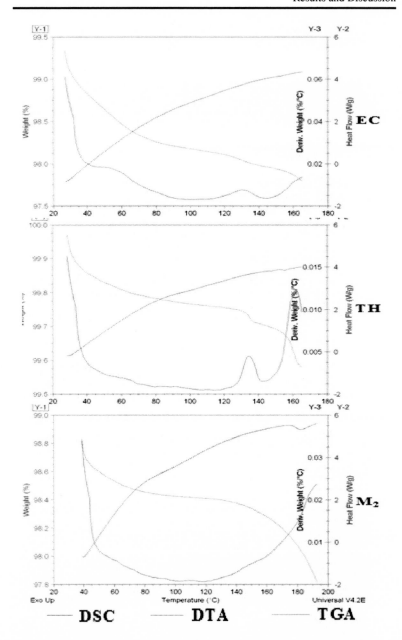

Figure 4.15: Thermograms of tramadol hydrochloride, ethylcellulose and M_2 formulation

4.3. Preparation and Physicochemical Characterization of Diclofenac sodium Microparticles

This study provides chemistry of EC, physics of DS release through particle wall and use of microparticles in life sciences. DS-EC microparticles were prepared by non-solvent addition phase separation method involving toluene as solvent and petroleum benzin as non-solvent. Time required for microencapsulation by this method is almost one hour that is less than most of the other microencapsulation methods.

4.3.1. Embedment Efficiency and Microparticle Size

Microparticle drug embedment efficiency was found to increase by increasing polymer drug ratio from 1:1 to 1:3. Microparticles with 1:3 ratio were found to have optimum embedded drug. No significant change in drug embedment efficiency was observed with further increase in EC concentration (Table 4.11). The results indicate that embedment efficiency also affected particle size. Large size microparticles were observed with higher embedment efficiency. This might be due to increase in system viscosity with increase in EC concentration. Increased viscosity caused the adherence of higher number of individual particles and resulted in larger microparticles. These results are comparable with previous results (Sajeev et al., 2002; Biju et al., 2004) where an increase in polymer viscosity resulted in larger microparticles. Magnetic stirring speed and its duration did not affect embedment efficiency. However, prolonged stirring at higher speed produced microparticles of smaller size.

4.3.2. Yield Efficiency

Good yield efficiency (~90%) was achieved for all batches. Moreover, an increased polymer concentration increased yield insignificantly (Table 4.11). Sajeev et al., (2002) have also presented similar results.

4.3.3. Scanning Electron Microscopy

According to SEM results, microparticles were irregular in shape with deep cracks in

Table 4.11: Physical evaluation of diclofenac sodium microparticles

Formulations	Drug: Polymer ratio	Embedment efficiency (%)	yield efficiency (M ± S.D)%	Size (Mean Diameter) (M ± S.D) μm	$t_{60\%}$ (M ± S.D) (h)
M_1	1:1	88.94	89.87 ± 1.29	389.62 ± 14.15	1.70
M_2	1:2	90.04	90.57 ± 1.15	410.94 ± 09.64	2.06
M_3	1:3	90.89	90.23 ± 1.24	442.19 ± 18.15	2.33

their rough surface (Figure 4.16).

4.3.4. Fourier Transform Infrared Spectroscopy

FTIR spectra showed no degradation of drug during microencapsulation. Amino peak N-H stretching and C-Cl stretching appeared at 3320 and 768 that represented DS in EC. Aromatic peak C-H stretching at 3020 confirmed EC. The nature of peaks did not vary in pure and microparticle form that showed no interaction between drug and polymer (Figure 4.17).

4.3.5. X-ray Diffractometry

X-ray powder diffraction patterns of DS revealed its crystalline form. Where as, DS crystallinity decreased in the form of its microparticles. This decrease in crystallinity is supported by diffractograms given in Figure 4.18.

4.3.6. Thermal Analysis

As shown in thermograms (Figure 4.19), a sharp DTA peak was observed between 50 to 100°C in thermograms of DS and M_2. In case of DS-EC microparticles DSC curve, a exothermic peak was observed at 70°C but with much reduced sharpness indicating slight variation in crystallinity of drug in the form of microparticles. No sudden change in thermal behavior of DS in both states indicated the absence of any possible drug-polymer interaction. Thermal analysis therefore, revealed good stability of DS in the form of DS-EC microparticles.

4.3.7. Micromeritic Properties

Rheological studies are described in Table 4.12. Pure DS and its microparticles showed identical bulk and tapped densities. However, in terms of angle of repose and compressibility index, flow properties of microparticles were better than pure drug. Thus, microparticles had improved packability and flow characteristics i.e. ease of handling, compared to pure DS crystals.

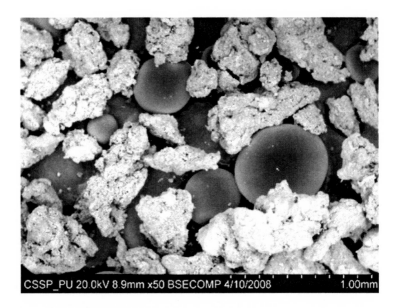

Figure 4.16: Scanning electron micrographs of diclofenac sodium microparticles (M_2)

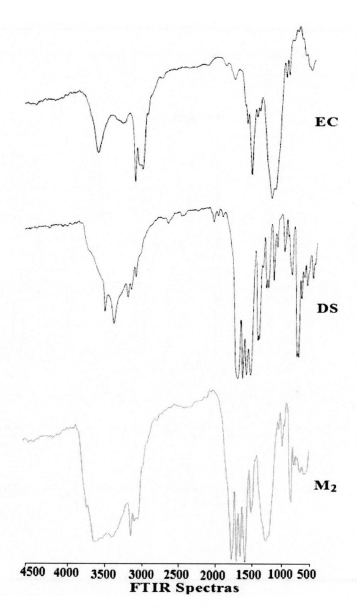

Figure 4.17: FTIR spectras of diclofenac sodium, ethylcellulose and formulation M_2

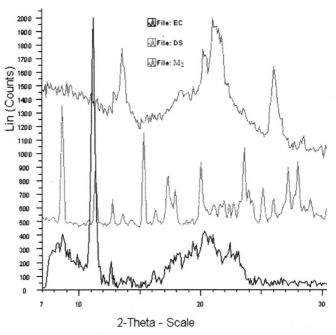

Figure 4.18: X-ray diffractometry of ethylcellulose, diclofenac sodium and
formulation M₂

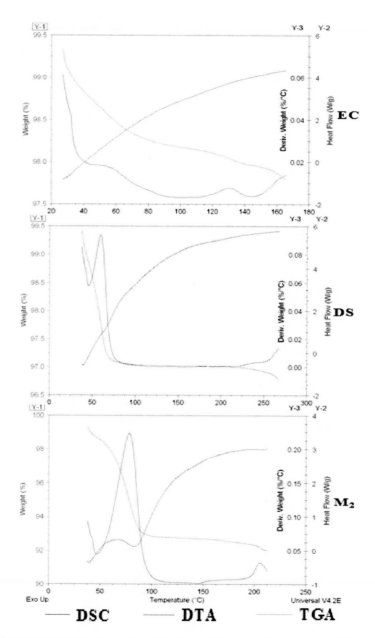

Figure 4.19: Thermograms of formulation M₂, diclofenac sodium and ethylcellulose

Table 4.12: Rheological properties of diclofenac sodium microparticles

Formulations	Bulk density (g/ml)	Taped density (g/ml)	Compressibility index (%)	Hausner's ratio	Angle of repose ($\theta°$)
M_1	0.30	0.24	12.43	1.22	19.78
M_2	0.24	0.29	11.09	1.15	22.47
M_3	0.28	0.27	12.93	1.19	21.72

4.3.8. In vitro Dissolution Studies

Figure 4.20 shows in vitro release pattern of various DS-EC microparticle formulations. Polymer concentration governed the drug release from microparticles. 90% drug release from pure DS raw material, M_1, M_2 and M_3 was achieved in 0.12, 1.70, 2.06 and 2.33 hours, respectively. It revealed sustained release behavior of microparticles. Microparticles with low polymer concentration released drug quickly. As mentioned earlier, microparticles with low polymer concentration were smaller in size which provided a larger surface area for faster drug release. This result is in accordance with modified Noyes-Whitney equation (Ansel et al., 1999):

$$(dc/dt) = kS\ (Cs - Ct)$$

Where dc/dt is the rate of dissolution, k is the dissolution rate constant, S is the surface area of dissolving body and Cs – Ct is the concentration gradient. Above mentioned results also revealed that the nature of drug changed from crystalline to amorphous during microencapsulation. Since, the amorphous form of a drug is usually more soluble than the crystalline form. Therefore, the release of drug from microparticles is quicker than other dosage form that satisfies immediate therapeutic effect.

The microparticles were also evaluated by using mathematical kinetic models i.e. difference & similarity factors and one way ANOVA plus Post-Hoc Tests. According to Duncan test, $t_{60\%}$ of all microparticle batches lied in the same homogenous group ($M_1=M_2=M_3$) whereas Tukey H.S.D. similarized $t_{60\%}$ of M_1 and M_2, and differentiated them from that of M_3 but not significantly ($p>0.05$). According to difference factor (f_1) and similarity factor (f_2), the release profiles of following microparticle formulations were different from each other: M_1 VS M_3 as their $f_1>15.00$ and $f_2<50.00$. While M_1 VS M_2 and M_2 VS M_3 have $f_1<15.00$ and $f_2>50.00$ that indicated

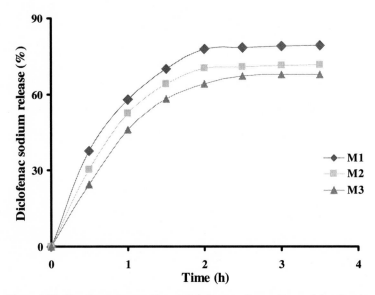

Figure 4.20: The dissolution profiles of diclofenac sodium microparticles showing the effect of polymer concentration. Each data point is a mean of three values.

the mutual similarity of the compared release profiles but to a very less extent. With a decreasing core to wall ratio, the velocity of drug release decreases. It can be assumed that with decreasing core to wall ratios, wall thickness of microparticles increases which then slows down the diffusion of dissolution medium into the microparticles. The number of surface pores decreased with increasing polymer concentration (Al-Taani and Tashtoush, 2003; Barik et al., 2001).

Higuchi model best explained the drug release pattern i.e. release of drug is directly proportional to the square root of time. The value of R^2 was 0.973. Anomalous diffusion was the mechanism of drug release from microparticles. The application of release profiles to the Hixson-Crowell equation indicated a change in surface area and diameter of the formulation with progressive dissolution of matrix as a function of time.

4.3.9. Estimation of Swelling and Erosion of Microparticles

M_2 undergoes swelling and erosion continuously with time (h) after putting into dissolution apparatus as clear from Figure 4.21. It is the reason for slow release of drug from microcapsule matrix. It also attests anomalous diffusion of DS from microparticles.

4.3.10. Stability Studies

No significant variation was observed in the drug contents of microparticles stored in above mentioned conditions after eight week chemical study. Drug embedment efficiency and the release profiles did not vary during this period. Thus, DS-EC microparticles showed good stability in these conditions.

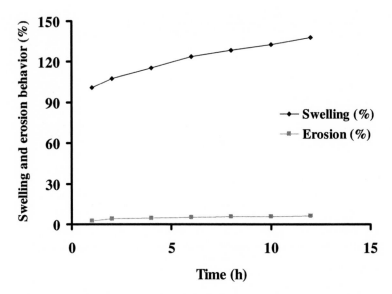

Figure 4.21: Erosion (%) and swelling (%) behavior of M_2. Each data point is a mean ± S.D. of three values.

4.4. In-vitro Analysis for the Suitability and Efficiency of a Microencapsulation Technique for Model Drugs having Different Water Solubilities

The non-solvent addition coacervation technique was applied to prepare SS, DS and TH microcapsules. Toluene was used as a solvent for EC, whereas SS, DS and TH are toluene insoluble drugs. Petroleum ether was used as a non-solvent to induce coacervation. EC was used as a wall-forming material on account of its safety, stability, hydrophobicity and compact film forming nature among water insoluble polymers (Rowe et al., 2004). The study was focused on the effect of drug polymer ratio and comparison of encapsulated SS, DS and TH (an intra-drug and inter drug comparison of their formulation characteristics).

4.4.1. Physicochemical Evaluation of Microparticles

The investigations were analyzed for their encapsulation efficiency. This study demonstrated that the encapsulation efficiency is influenced by core to wall ratio as shown in Table 4.13. With increasing polymer ratio, more particles of drug are coated with polymer which leads to a higher encapsulation efficiency (Singh and Robinson, 1990; Breghausen et al., 2002). However, this increase is not significant ($p > 0.05$) statistically. On the other hand, a decreasing order of encapsulation efficiency of these drugs was found following: SS > DS > TH ($P>0.05$). This insignificant difference in encapsulation efficiency of different drugs may be attributed to their respective solubility in solvent and non-solvent.

It is evident from Table 4.13 that increase in EC concentration caused a slight increase in production yield of microcapsules ($p>0.05$). Where as, percentage production yield was in decreasing order of these drugs SS>TH>DS ($p<0.05$). Some portion of DS dissolved in toluene during the encapsulation process. This DS wasted when toluene was separated from microcapsules by filtration. This reason may account for less production yield of DS microcapsules, accordingly.

Table 4.13: Evaluation of Physical Characteristics of Tramadol hydrochloride, Salbutamol sulphate and Diclofenac sodium Microcapsules

Formulations	Drug: Polymer ratio	Entrapment (%)	Production yield (M ± S.D)%	Size (Mean Diameter) (M ± S.D) μm	$t_{60\%}$ (M ± S.D) (hrs)
M_{TH1}	1:1	97.23	97.14 ± 1.47	73.02 ± 24.39	0.86
M_{TH2}	1:2	97.91	96.43 ± 1.32	75.71 ± 18.67	1.13
M_{TH3}	1:3	98.07	97.91 ± 1.36	76.23 ± 10.75	1.52
M_{SS1}	1:1	96.68	97.48 ± 1.21	68.37 ± 19.31	0.85
M_{SS2}	1:2	96.98	98.19 ± 1.20	70.04 ± 27.15	1.44
M_{SS3}	1:3	97.83	98.33 ± 1.37	72.01 ± 19.71	2.93
M_{DS1}	1:1	88.94	89.87 ± 1.29	89.62 ± 14.15	1.70
M_{DS2}	1:2	90.04	90.57 ± 1.15	90.94 ± 09.64	2.06
M_{DS3}	1:3	90.89	90.23 ± 1.24	92.19 ± 18.15	2.33

M_{TH}= Tramadol hydrochloride microcapsules
M_{SS} = Salbutamol sulphate microcapsules
M_{DS}= Diclofenac sodium microcapsules

The microcapsules were aggregated, whitish and irregular in shape (Figure 4.22). For TH, SS and DS, it was found that there was an increasing trend in particle size with an increase in polymer concentration ($p > 0.05$, Table 4.13). This increase in size can be attributed to the increased aggregation of EC particles with an increase in polymer concentration (Amperiadou and Georgarakis, 1995; Sajeev et al., 2002). On the other side, these drugs can be placed in decreasing order of their microcapsule size as: TH > DS > SS ($p < 0.05$). However, the reason of this difference in mean particle size of various drugs requires further investigation.

4.4.2. Physical Characterization of Tabletted Microcapsules

Physical attributes of tablets i.e. physical appearance, tablet hardness, weight variation, tablet thickness, friability and drug content uniformity of tabletted microcapsules were found to be satisfactory. Tablet hardness varied between 7.9 ± 1.0 to 9.2 ± 1.3 kg/cm^2 and friability was less than 0.5% (w/w). The designed tablets showed low weight variation ($< \pm 3.0\%$). The average thickness was 3.87 to 3.89 mm. The results fulfilled the requirements of B.P. (2004).

4.4.3. In vitro Dissolution Studies

4.4.3.1. Model independent approaches

The designed microcapsules and tabletted microcapsules were characterized for their release behavior in double distilled water and were evaluated by mathematical kinetic membrane within water filled pores (Breghausen et al., 2002). Thus, the release of TH, SS and DS from their respective microcapsules was influenced by the core to wall ratio as given in Figure 4.23 & 4.24. Comparison between dissolution profiles of TH microcapsules showed that 60% release of drug from its respective microcapsules was achieved in almost 0.86 (M_{TH1}), 1.13 (M_{TH2}) and 1.52 (M_{TH3}) hours, when drug polymer ratio was 1:1, 1:2 and 1:3, respectively. For the same drug polymer ratio,

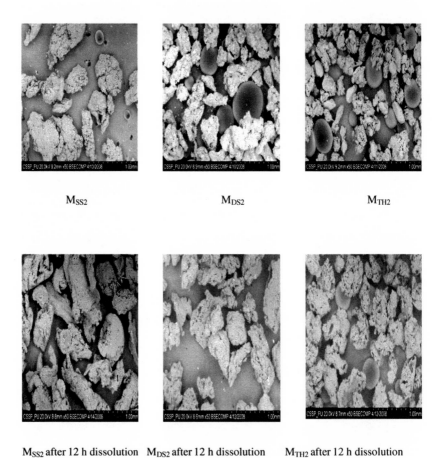

M_{SS2} M_{DS2} M_{TH2}

M_{SS2} after 12 h dissolution M_{DS2} after 12 h dissolution M_{TH2} after 12 h dissolution

Figure 4.22: Scanning electron micrographs of various microencapsulated
formulations

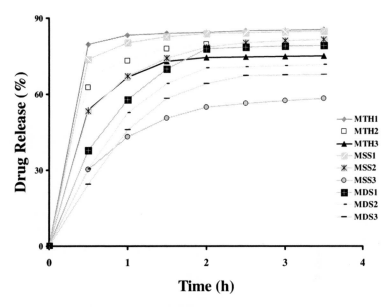

Figure 4.23: Zero order plots between average rate of dissolution of TH, SS & DS microcapsules and time (h) in double distilled water

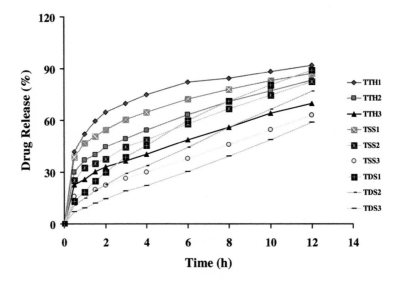

Figure 4.24: Zero order plots between average rate of dissolution of TH, SS & DS tablets and time (h) in double distilled water

60% release of SS was achieved after 0.85, 1.44 and 2.93 hours. Similarly, 60% release of DS was achieved after 1.70, 2.06 and 2.33 hours, when drug polymer ratio was 1:1, 1:2 and 1:3. According to Duncan test, the $t_{60\%}$ of all batches of the microcapsules lied in the same homogenous group (1:1=1:2=1:3) (p>0.05) whereas Tukey H.S.D. similarized $t_{60\%}$ of 1:1 & 1:2 and differentiated them from that of 1:3 insignificantly. On the other hand, Duncan test places these drugs in the following setting based on their $t_{60\%}$ of microcapsules and tabletted microcapsules: TH=SS=DS (p>0.05). Tukey test differentiate DS from TH and SS insignificantly on the basis of their $t_{60\%}$ of microcapsules and tabletted microcapsules. This little difference could be attributed to the nature and solubility differences of these drugs. According to difference factor (f_1) and similarity factor (f_2), release profiles of following pairs of microcapsule batches are similar to each other: M_{TH1} Vs M_{SS1}, M_{TH2} Vs M_{SS2}, M_{TH3} Vs M_{SS3} as their $f_1 < 15.00$ and $f_2 > 50.00$. While other compared batches of microcapsules have $f_1 > 15.00$ and $f_2 < 50.00$ that indicates the mutual dissimilarity of the compared release profiles. With a decreasing core to wall ratio, the drug release slows down, the wall thickness of microcapsules increases which then slows down the diffusion of dissolution medium into the microcapsules. The number of surface pores decreased with increasing polymer concentration (p<0.05) (Amperiadou and Georgarakis, 1995; Sajeev et al., 2002; Breghausen et al., 2002).

The observed in-vitro drug release profiles from TH and SS microparticles were biphasic: an initial rapid drug release phase (burst) was followed by the slow and prolonged phase. The burst effect may be beneficial because a high initial release produces an instant effect which can be subsequently maintained for a prolonged period by a slower but continuous release of these drugs. The rank order of drug: polymer ratios for percentage drug burst was: 1:1>1:2>1:3, as visible from plots 4.23

and 4.24. Whereas, more burst effect is seen in the release profiles of TH than that of SS. The rapid initial phase of release was thought to occur mainly by dissolution and diffusion of drug entrapped close to or at the surface of microparticles. The second and slower release phase was thought to involve diffusion of drug entrapped within inner part of the polymer matrix by means of aqueous channels of a network of pores. It has been already reported that an initial burst effect in release profile was observed especially (a) when the drug solubility is high, (b) loading dose in the polymeric matrix is large and (c) lack of critical polymer concentration.

Additionally, when polymer concentration is low, the hydrated polymeric matrix would be highly porous leading to rapid diffusion of drug from the polymeric matrix (Erden and Celebi, 1996; Singh and Robinson, 1990).

It was observed that initial rate of release for the first 1hour was high (46-52%) for TH and SS tabletted microcapsules when drug polymer ratio was 1:1 but release was slow in case of DS tabletted microcapsules. However, the release in the long term was slower from tablets with higher drug polymer ratio (1:2, 1:3) as in both cases; drug release was extended beyond 12 hours for all the three drugs. Moreover, the initial release rate from SS and TH tabletted microcapsules was somewhat high due to burst effect; the incorporation of loading dose appeared unnecessary (Figure 4.23). Depending on $t_{60\%}$ of tabletted microcapsules, Post-Hoc (Duncan) test distributes various drug polymer ratios (Irrespective of drug) in the order of: 1:3>1:1=1:2. In case of tablets, the compared formulations i.e. T_{TH1} Vs T_{SS1}, T_{TH2} Vs T_{SS2}, T_{TH3} Vs T_{SS3} and T_{SS3} Vs T_{DS3} have $f1<15.00$ and $f2>50.00$, so both release profiles of each pair are almost similar to each other while others have $f1>15.00$ and $f2<50.00$ which shows dissimilarity between release profiles of each pair.

4.4.3.2. Model dependent approaches

To get meaningful information, the whole drug release profiles were evaluated kinetically and the best fit of release profiles to the zero order, first order, Higuchi, Hixson-Crowell and Korsmeyer-Peppas models was investigated. Model with the highest co-efficient of determination was judged to be a more appropriate model for the dissolution data. The release profiles from all the microcapsules were best explained by Higuchi model due to the highest linearity, followed by zero order and first order. It suggests that the drug release is controlled by diffusion of drug through pores and not through swollen polymer. TH and SS and T_{DS1} tablets also followed same kinetic model. However, in case of T_{DS2} & T_{DS3}, best fit kinetic model found was Zero order. From Korsmeyer-Peppas model, it is found that the mode of release from all microcapsules and tabletted microcapsules was anomalous (non-Fickian, a combination of the diffusion and erosion mechanism) diffusion except T_{DS2} and T_{DS3} that showed a non-Fickian super case II as shown in Table 4.14 & 4.15.

The application of release profiles to the Hixson-Crowell equation indicated a change in surface area and diameter of formulation with progressive dissolution of matrix as a function of time.

4.4.4. Batch Reproducibility and Stability on Storage

No significant ($p > 0.05$) difference was observed in the release profiles of different batches of tabletted microcapsules, indicating that the manufacturing process used was reliable and reproducible ($p > 0.05$, $f_1 < 0.29$, $f_2 > 99.71$). Also, the release kinetics remained unaltered for up to three months of storage, and there were no changes in the tablet characteristics suggesting that TH, SS and DS were stable in the tabletted microcapsules for the above mentioned period.

Table 4.14: Release Rate Parameters [Y-equation (Y=aX + b), Determination Co-efficient (R^2), Correlation Co-efficient (r) and Release Exponent (n)] for Release Data after Fitting of the whole Release Profiles of TH, SS and DS from their Respective Microcapsules into Different Mathematical Models.

Formulations	Size (Mean Diameter) (M ± S.D.) μm	Zero Order		First Order		Higuchi		Hixson-Crowell		Korsmeyer-peppa		
		Y-equation	R^2	Y-equation	R^2	Y-equation	R^2	Y-equation	R^2	Y-equation	R^2	n
M_{TH1}	73.02 ± 24.3	15.03x + 47.07	0.38	0.7509x + 2.5612	0.35	5.0925x + 26.382	0.67	-0.4061x + 3.4993	0.44	0.697x + 3.5552	0.09	0.70
M_{TH2}	75.71 ± 18.6	16.241x + 38.564	0.51	0.7702x + 2.4447	0.38	5.1808x + 19.18	0.79	-0.4322x + 3.8242	0.61	0.7708x + 3.4387	0.11	0.77
M_{TH3}	76.23 ± 10.7	15.65x + 34.185	0.55	0.768x + 2.3725	0.39	4.9241x + 16.135	0.82	-0.3873x + 3.95	0.63	0.7922x + 3.3529	0.12	0.79
M_{SS1}	68.37 ± 19.3	15.723x + 44.274	0.43	0.76x + 2.5255	0.36	5.1976x + 23.829	0.72	-0.4332x + 3.6203	0.52	0.7259x + 3.5222	0.09	0.73
M_{SS2}	70.04 ± 27.1	17.965x + 33.09	0.63	0.7979x + 2.3583	0.41	5.4628x + 14.121	0.88	-0.4858x + 3.9978	0.75	0.8469x + 3.3658	0.14	0.85
M_{SS3}	72.01 ± 19.7	13.977x + 19.367	0.73	0.7747x + 2.0498	0.46	13.977x + 19.367	0.73	-0.2952x + 4.3068	0.79	0.8933x + 2.9953	0.18	0.89
M_{DS1}	89.62 ± 14.1	19.792x + 25.411	0.73	0.8413x + 2.2026	0.47	5.7361x + 7.1174	0.93	-0.5164x + 4.1886	0.82	0.9839x + 3.2231	0.19	0.98
M_{DS2}	90.94 ± 09.6	18.252x + 21.943	0.74	0.8368x + 2.109	0.48	5.2603x + 5.3435	0.93	-0.4337x + 4.2543	0.80	1.0096x + 3.1099	0.21	1.01
M_{DS3}	92.19 ± 18.1	18.104x + 17.751	0.79	0.8533x + 1.9929	0.52	5.0956x + 2.4133	0.95	-0.413x + 4.3459	0.85	1.0733x + 2.9934	0.24	1.07

Table 4.15: Release Rate Parameters [Y-equation (Y=aX + b), Determination Co-efficient (R^2), Correlation Co-efficient (r) and Release Exponent (n)] for Release Data after fitting of the whole release profiles of TH, SS and DS from their respective Tabletted Microcapsules into Different Mathematical Models.

Formulations	Zero Order		First Order		Higuchi		Hixson-Crowell		Korsmeyer-peppa		
	Y-equation	R^2	Y-equation	R^2	Y-equation	R^2	Y-equation	R^2	Y-equation	R^2	n
T_{TH1}	5.1338x + 42.175	0.63	0.1584x + 3.1597	0.25	2.9257x + 23.408	0.87	-0.1729x + 3.8694	0.94	0.6116x + 3.209	0.25	0.61
T_{TH2}	5.2952x + 26.849	0.83	0.1733x + 2.8401	0.33	2.7963x + 10.609	0.97	-0.1434x + 4.2211	0.99	0.6587x + 2.9049	0.32	0.66
T_{TH3}	4.6454x + 18.648	0.89	0.1773x + 2.582	0.38	2.3851x + 5.3577	0.98	-0.107x + 4.3589	0.99	0.6691x + 2.653	0.36	0.67
T_{SS1}	5.0685x + 35.772	0.71	0.1615x + 3.0436	0.27	2.795x + 18.56	0.91	-0.1517x + 4.0255	0.98	0.6137x + 3.1039	0.26	0.61
T_{SS2}	5.468x + 22.117	0.89	0.182x + 2.712	0.37	2.8179x + 6.3263	0.99	-0.143x + 4.3204	0.99	0.6914x + 2.7802	0.36	0.69
T_{SS3}	4.418x + 11.164	0.95	4.418x + 11.164	0.48	2.1794x – 0.2247	0.98	-0.0937x + 4.4887	0.99	0.7139x + 2.3484	0.45	0.71
T_{DS1}	6.9956x + 12.337	0.96	0.2267x + 2.3579	0.53	3.4655x – 5.9006	0.99	-0.1903x + 4.5455	0.99	0.8969x + 2.4054	0.56	0.90
T_{DS2}	5.9016x + 8.298	0.98	0.2253x + 2.1461	0.58	2.8692x – 6.322	0.98	-0.1369x + 4.5692	0.99	0.878x + 2.2073	0.59	0.88
T_{DS3}	4.5179x + 4.0216	0.99	0.2292x + 1.7665	0.67	2.1557x – 6.5968	0.95	-0.0906x + 4.607	0.99	0.888x + 1.8342	0.68	0.89

4.4.5. Drug Interaction Study

The UV spectra of pure drug solution and solution prepared for the determination of drug entrapment efficiency of drug loaded microcapsules were of the same kind. The λ_{max} of pure TH, SS and DS was observed at 271 nm, 276 nm and 276 nm, respectively.

Some characteristic and prominent peaks of these drugs were observed in FTIR spectrum. The spectrum of the formulations showed all the characteristic peaks of relevant drugs (Figure 4.25). Thus, both spectroscopy results denied any strong interaction of EC with these drugs when encapsulated into EC coats.

Thermal analysis showed good stability of all three drugs in the form of microparticles (Figure 4.26). The characteristic, well-recognizable thermal profile of drugs in a specific temperature range was observed. The same thermal behavior was observed in case of their microparticles but with the loss of its sharp appearance that indicated a significant reduction of drug crystallinity in the polymer matrix. It indicated the absence of any strong chemical interaction between drug and polymer. X-ray diffractometry revealed amorphous and crystalline nature of pure drugs, respectively as shown in diffractograms (Figure 4.27). However, a decrease in the signal intensity i.e. crystallinity of drugs was observed in microparticle form as compared to pure components.

4.4.6. Estimation of Swelling and Erosion of Tabletted Microparticles

The optimum formulations undergoes swelling and erosion continuously with time (h) after putting into dissolution apparatus as clear from Figure 4.28. This phenomenon is responsible for gradual release of drug from tabletted microcapsule matrix. It also confirms anomalous diffusion of drug from these three tabletted microparticles.

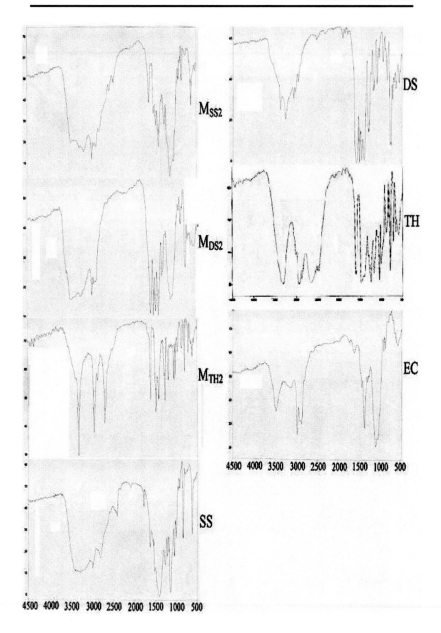

Figure 4.25: FTIR spectras of diclofenac sodium, salbutamol sulphate, tramadol hydrochloride, ethylcellulose, M_{SS2}, M_{DS2} and M_{TH2}.

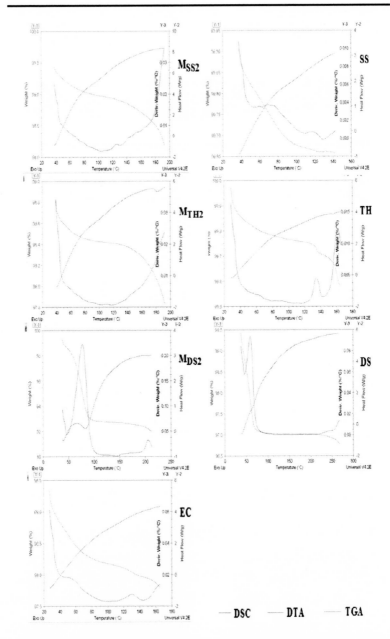

Figure 4.26: Thermograms of diclofenac sodium, salbutamol sulphate, tramadol hydrochloride, ethylcellulose, M_{SS2}, M_{DS2} and M_{TH2}.

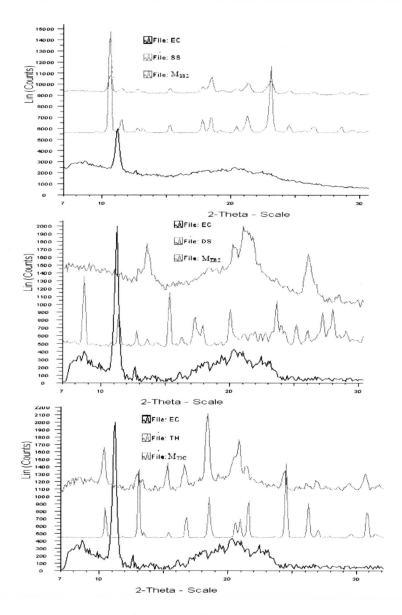

Figure 4.27: X-ray diffractograms of diclofenac sodium, salbutamol sulphate, tramadol hydrochloride, ethylcellulose, formulation M_{SS2}, M_{DS2} and M_{TH2}.

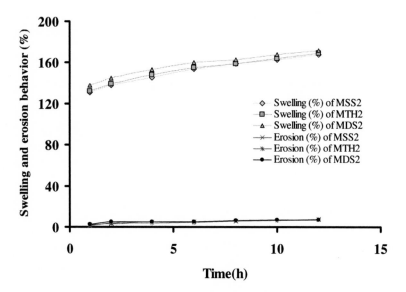

Figure 4.28: Erosion (%) and swelling (%) behavior of microparticles of diclofenac sodium, salbutamol sulphate, tramadol hydrochloride, ethylcellulose, M_{SS2}, M_{DS2} and M_{TH2}. Each data point is a mean ± S.D. of three values.

4.5. A Comparative Study of Various Microencapsulation Techniques: Effect of Polymer Viscosity on Microcapsule Characteristics

Ethylcellulose was used as a shell material due to of its safety, stability, hydrophobicity and perfect film forming nature among lipophilic polymers (Rowe et al., 2003). The study was focused on the effect of EC viscosity grades, drug polymer ratios and the type of microencapsulation technique on drug contents and release profiles.

Salbutamol sulphate containing microcapsules were prepared by various methods as mentioned earlier. Coacervation Thermal change was the most rapid of the three methods. The approximate time consumed for preparation of microcapsules by SE, CTC and CNSA were 7 h, 10 h and 4 h, respectively.

The microcapsules were aggregated, whitish and irregular in shape (Figure 4.29 A, B and C). Table 4.16 shows a comparison of mean particle size of microcapsules prepared by these three techniques. The smallest particle size was achieved by SE technique. Insignificantly larger size microparticles, prepared by other methods, may be due to an aggregation of individual microparticles which may also account for their slow release of SS due to slow penetration of dissolution medium into aggregated microcapsules (Sajeev et al 2002).

Table 4.16 depicts excellent percentage production yield with good encapsulation efficiencies for all the formulations. Out of three methods, CNSA showed highest percentage production yield and encapsulation efficiency which can be justified on the basis of less solubility of SS in the solvent (toluene).

Rheological properties of all formulations are expressed in terms of bulk density, taped density, compressibility index, Hausner's ratio and angle of repose (Table 4.17). It was observed that bulk density decreased with increase in drug polymer ratio. Present results are in close agreement with those reported by Shariff et al., (2007)

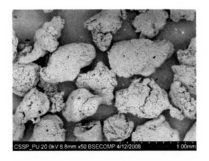

Figure 4.29A: Scanning electron micrographs of M_2

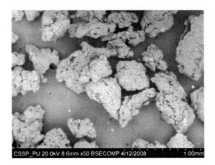

Figure 4.29B: Scanning electron micrographs of M_5

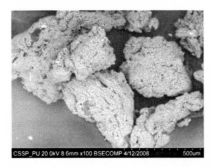

Figure 4.29C: Scanning electron micrographs of M_8

Figure 4.16: Physical characteristics of microcapsules prepared by coacervation- thermal change, coacervation- non-solvent addition and o/o emulsion solvent evaporation technique

Formulations	Drug: Polymer ratio	Entrapment (%)	Production yield $(M \pm S.D)\%$	Size(Mean Diameter) $(M \pm S.D)$ μm	Hydration Rate (%)	$t_{60\%}$ $(M \pm S.D)$ (hrs)
$M_1^\dagger$	1:1	95.23	94.38 ± 0.95	79.84 ± 09.58	157.95	0.34
$M_2^\dagger$	1:2	95.91	94.97 ± 0.83	80.51 ± 13.54	167.39	0.93
$M_3^\dagger$	1:3	97.07	95.37 ± 1.02	82.97 ± 10.18	169.65	2.16
$M_4^{\maltese}$	1:1	96.68	97.48 ± 1.21	68.37 ± 19.31	176.19	0.35
$M_5^{\maltese}$	1:2	96.98	98.19 ± 1.20	70.04 ± 27.15	155.12	0.94
$M_6^{\maltese}$	1:3	97.83	98.33 ± 1.37	72.01 ± 19.71	176.28	2.16
$M_7^{\bullet}$	1:1	86.34	87.91 ± 1.34	43.57 ± 18.28	183.64	0.23
$M_8^{\bullet}$	1:2	89.84	89.27 ± 1.19	45.98 ± 11.54	181.65	0.86
$M_9^{\bullet}$	1:3	92.78	88.93 ± 1.13	48.04 ± 21.07	169.52	2.01
$M_{10}^{\maltese}$	1:2	97.06	98.17 ± 1.40	70.91 ± 18.45	159.87	1.19
$M_{11}^{\maltese}$	1:2	97.23	98.51 ± 1.13	71.12 ± 32.11	163.27	1.72

$\dagger$ Microcapsules prepared by Coacervation- Thermal Change Technique

$\maltese$ Microcapsules prepared by Coacervation- Non-solvent Addition Technique

$\bullet$ Microcapsules prepared by O/O Emulsion Solvent Evaporation Technique

Table 4.17: Rheological properties of $M_1 - M_{11}$ microcapsule formulations

Formulations	Bulk density (g/ml)	Taped density (g/ml)	Compressibility index (%)	Hausner's ratio	Angle of repose
M_1	0.21	0.23	11.0	1.16	21.87°
M_2	0.26	0.31	12.87	1.09	23.94°
M_3	0.30	0.33	10.39	1.29	27.45°
M_4	0.29	0.29	13.15	1.03	28.68°
M_5	0.24	0.26	13.62	1.17	25.13°
M_6	0.18	0.21	10.08	1.46	29.65°
M_7	0.23	0.34	09.12	1.90	22.08°
M_8	0.19	0.39	12.82	1.13	19.71°
M_9	0.23	0.19	11.35	1.24	26.58°
M_{10}	0.29	0.30	13.76	1.25	29.27°
M_{11}	0.31	0.28	13.87	1.31	31.33°

who have also reported that bulk density increased when polymer concentration was decreased. Compressibility index of all six formulations is below 15% indicating excellent flow properties. Hausner's ratio for all formulations was below 1.29 again indicating free flow of all formulations of microcapsules and similarly angle of repose for all formulations are below 30° indicating once again free flowing nature of microcapsules.

4.5.1. Model Analysis and Statistics

4.5.1.1. Model independent approaches

The designed microcapsules were characterized for their release behavior in double distilled water and were evaluated by mathematical kinetic models, the difference & similarity factors and one way ANOVA plus Post-Hoc Test. EC is a non-water soluble polymer. Therefore, the release of water soluble drugs is mainly driven by permeation of drug through hydrophobic polymer membrane within water filled pores (Breghausen et al., 2002). Thus, the release of salbutamol sulpahte from its microcapsules was influenced by core to wall ratio as given graphically in Figure 4.30. The application of analysis of variance elaborated that the change in method of microencapsulation affected the release of SS from its microcapsules (p>0.05).

Comparison between $t_{50\%}$ showed that the release of salbutamol sulpahte from its CNSA microcapsules was the most rapid followed by from that of CTC and SE, respectively. CNSA involves slow solidification of microcapsules with comparatively less pores and fractures in EC shells which allow slow penetration of dissolution medium. This is the reason of slow release of SS from its microcapsules as compared with that of CTC and SE. The rapid solidification of CTC microcapsules causes increased fractures in EC shells followed by comparatively fast SS release. Whereas

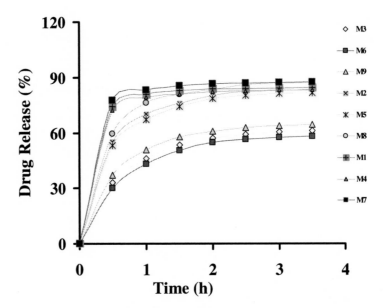

Figure 4.30: The dissolution profiles of salbutamol sulphate microcapsules in distilled water showing the effect of different techniques of microencapsulation on its dissolution behavior.

the $t_{50\%}$ of SE microcapsules lies intermediate to that of other two. According to Duncan test, the $t_{50\%}$ of all batches of microcapsules of same drug-polymer ratio lied in the same homogenous group (CTC=CNSA=SE) ($p>0.05$). According to difference factor (f_1) and similarity factor (f_2), the release profiles of all batches of microcapsules of same drug-polymer ratio prepared by different techniques are similar to each other as their $f_1 < 15.00$ and $f_2 > 50.00$ (p > 0.05). With a decreasing core to wall ratio, the velocity of drug release decreases. It can be assumed that with decreasing core to wall ratios, the wall thickness of microcapsules increases which then slows down the diffusion of dissolution medium into microcapsules. The number of surface pores decreased with increasing polymer concentration (p<0.05) (Sajeev et al., 2002; Breghausen et al., 2002). However, the results indicate that release behavior is arbitrarily affected by particle size of microcapsules in the present work.

The observed in-vitro drug release profiles from salbutamol sulpahte microparticles were biphasic: an initial rapid drug release phase (burst) was followed by slow and prolonged phase. The burst effect may be beneficial because a high initial release produces an instant effect which can subsequently be maintained for a prolonged period by a slower but continuous release of drug. The rank order of drug:polymer ratios for percentage drug burst was: 1:1>1:2>1:3, as visible from plots. The rapid initial phase of release was thought to occur mainly by dissolution and diffusion of drug entrapped close to or at the surface of microparticles. The second and slower release phase was thought to involve the diffusion of drug entrapped within inner part of polymer matrix by means of aqueous channels of a network of pores. It has already been reported that an initial burst effect in release profile was observed especially when (a) the drug solubility is high, (b) loading dose in the polymeric matrix is large and (c) lack of critical polymer concentration. Additionally, when polymer concentration is low, the hydrated polymeric matrix would be highly porous leading to rapid diffusion of drug from polymeric matrix (Erden and Celebi, 1996; Singh and Robinson, 1990).

4.5.1.2. Model dependent approaches

To obtain appropriate information, the whole drug release data was evaluated using different kinetic models i.e. zero order, first order, Higuchi, Hixson-Crowell and Korsmeyer-Peppas models. The best fit of these models to the release profiles was investigated (Table 4.18). Model with the highest co-efficient of determination was accepted as more appropriate model for the present dissolution data. The release patterns from all the formulations were best explained by Higuchi square root model due to the highest linearity, followed by zero order and first order. It confirms that SS release occurs by diffusion through pores and not through the swollen matrix. Korsmeyer-Peppas model further verified the mode of SS release from all microparticles that was anomalous diffusion (Non-Fickian i.e. a combination of the diffusion and erosion mechanisms). The application of Hixson-Crowell equation to the release data indicated a change in surface area and diameter of microcapsules with progressive dissolution of polymer as a function of time.

4.5.2. Effect of Viscosity Grade on Encapsulated SS

Salbutamol sulphate microcapsules were prepared using three different viscosity grades of EC by coacervation-non solvent addition technique with no change in other experimental parameters. The effect of viscosity grades on SS release kinetics is shown in Figure 4.31. It was observed that higher the viscosity grade, slower was the SS release especially in the initial stage ($p < 0.05$). Duncan test places the release profiles of 10 cp and 22 cp in the same group other than that of 46 cp. It shows that there is a significant ($p < 0.05$) difference in SS release pattern for different viscosity grades of

Table 4.18: Release rate parameters [y-equation (Y=aX + b), determination co-efficient (r^2) and release exponent (n)] for release data after fitting of the whole release profiles of salbutamol sulpahte from its respective microcapsules into different mathematical models.

Formulations	Zero Order Y-equation	R^2	First Order Y-equation	R^2	Higuchi Y-equation	R^2	Hixson-Crowell Y-equation	R^2	Korsmeyer-peppa Y-equation	R^2	n
M_1	15.539x + 44.624	0.424	-0.3843x + 3.7599	0.547	39.993x + 24.177	0.708	-0.4243x + 3.6043	0.499	0.7211x + 3.5248	0.093	0.72
M_2	18.212x + 34.423	0.615	-0.44584x + 4.1116	0.808	43.092x + 14.961	0.869	-0.5065x + 3.9621	0.745	0.8431x + 3.3918	0.132	0.84
M_3	14.457x + 21.045	0.713	-0.2251x + 4.377	0.813	32.858x + 7.2019	0.929	-0.2952x + 4.3068	0.786	0.8933x + 2.9953	0.179	0.89
M_4	15.43x + 43.394	0.434	-0.3702x + 3.8117	0.560	39.505x + 23.335	0.717	-0.4141x + 3.654	0.511	0.7238x + 3.5059	0.095	0.72
M_5	17.961x + 33.105	0.626	-0.43312x + 4.1403	0.807	42.31x + 14.133	0.876	-0.4857x + 3.9973	0.748	0.8468x + 3.3659	0.134	0.85
M_6	13.977x + 19.367	0.727	-0.2251x + 4.377	0.813	31.571x + 6.2169	0.936	-0.2952x + 4.3068	0.786	0.8933x + 2.9953	0.179	0.89
M_7	16.048x + 46.244	0.423	-0.435x + 3.6912	0.571	41.3x + 25.13	0.706	-0.4617x + 3.5384	0.512	0.7237x + 3.5538	0.092	0.72
M_8	18.589x + 37.536	0.585	-0.5205x + 4.0314	0.799	44.535x + 17.015	0.846	-0.55x + 3.8696	0.727	0.8321x + 3.4465	0.125	0.83
M_9	14.881x + 23.667	0.681	-0.2607x + 4.3095	0.788	34.273x + 8.8797	0.911	-0.3315x + 4.2165	0.753	0.8625x + 3.1251	0.157	0.86
M_{10}	17.473x + 36.68	0.571	-0.4376x + 4.0471	0.764	42.102x + 17.103	0.836	-0.4838x + 3.8923	0.698	0.809x + 3.4227	0.120	0.81
M_{11}	14.807x + 25.452	0.650	-0.264x + 4.2766	0.759	34.537x + 10.222	0.891	-0.3334x + 4.175	0.723	0.8425x + 3.1653	0.148	0.84

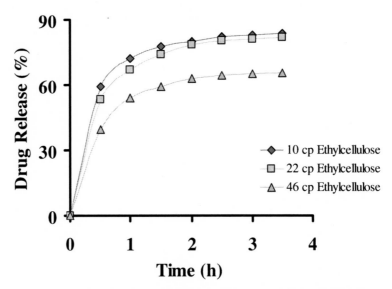

Figure 4.31: The dissolution profiles of salbutamol sulphate microcapsules in distilled water showing the effect of different viscosity grades of ethylcellulose (10 cp, 22 cp and 46 cp) on its dissolution behavior.

coating material. Comparison between $t_{50\%}$ showed that the release of salbutamol sulpahte from its M_5 microcapsules was the most rapid followed by from that of M_{10} and M_{11}, respectively. M_{10} microcapsules receive a thin polymer shell with comparatively more pores and fractures in EC shells which allow rapid penetration of dissolution medium. This is the reason of rapid release of SS from its microcapsules as compared with that of M_5 and M_{11}. The M_{11} microcapsules receive comparatively thick EC shells resulting comparatively slow SS release. Whereas the $t_{50\%}$ of M_5 microcapsules lies intermediate to that of other two. According to difference factor ($f1$) and similarity factor ($f2$), the release profiles of following pairs of microcapsule formulations are different from each other: M_{10} VS M_{11} and M_5 VS M_{11} as their $f1 >$ 15.00 and $f2 < 50.00$. While M_{10} VS M_5 has $f1 < 15.00$ and $f2 > 50.00$ that indicates mutual similarity of compared release profiles but to a very less extent (Singh, and Robinson, 1990; Uddin, Hawlader, and Zhu, 2001).

4.5.3. UV and FTIR Spectroscopy

The UV spectra of pure drug solution and solution prepared for the determination of drug entrapment efficiency of drug loaded microparticles were of the same kind. The λ_{max} of pure SS was observed at 276 nm on UV spectra of solution prepared for the determination of drug entrapment efficiency of SS loaded microparticles. Some characteristic and prominent peaks of SS were observed in FTIR spectrum. The spectrum of all microparticles showed amino, hydroxyl and aromatic stretchings at the same values as in that of pure SS which confirmed its presence. No significant alteration in the nature of peaks denied any strong SS-EC interaction when SS was encapsulated into EC coats. The relevant FTIR spectras are given in Figure 4.32.

4.5.4. Thermal Analysis

Thermal analysis showed good stability of SS in the form of all microparticles (Figure

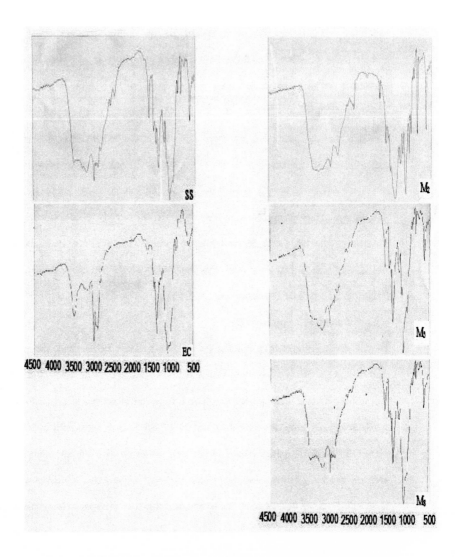

Figure 4.32: FTIR spectras of salbutamol sulphate, ethylcellulose, M_2, M_5 and M_8.

4.33). The characteristic, well-recognizable thermal profile of drug in a specific temperature range was observed. The same thermal behavior was observed in case of its all microparticles but with the loss of its sharp appearance that indicated a significant reduction of drug crystallinity in polymer matrix. It indicated the absence of any strong chemical interaction between drug and polymer.

4.5.5. X-ray Diffractometry

X-ray diffractometry revealed amorphous and crystalline nature of pure EC and SS, respectively as shown in diffractograms (Figure 4.34). However, a decrease in the signal intensity i.e. crystallinity of SS was observed in microparticle form as compared to pure components.

4.5.6. Estimation of swelling and Erosion of Tabletted Microparticles

The optimum formulations exhibited swelling and erosion continuously with time (h) after putting into dissolution apparatus as evident from Figure 4.35. This phenomenon is responsible for gradual release of drug from tabletted microcapsule matrix. It also confirms anomalous diffusion of SS from tabletted microparticles.

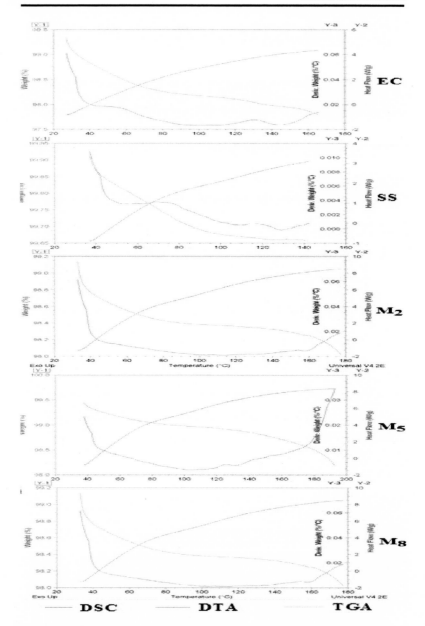

Figure 4.33: Thermograms of salbutamol sulphate, ethylcellulose, formulations M_2, M_5 and M_8.

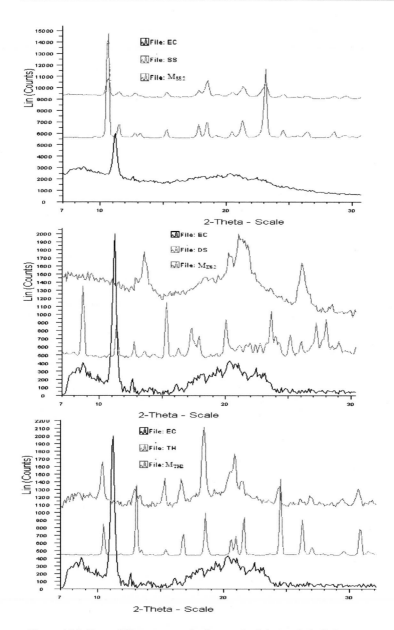

Figure 4.34: X-ray diffractograms of salbutamol sulphate, ethylcellulose, formulation M_2, M_5 and M_8.

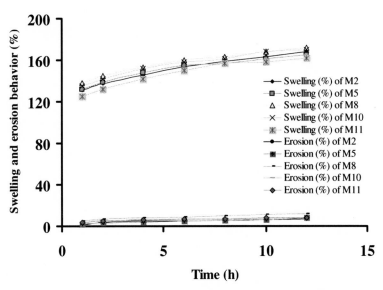

Figure 4.35: Swelling (%) and erosion (%) behavior of various formulations

4.6. Optimization and Validation of a New and Sensitive Reverse Phase HPLC Method with Fluorescent Detection for the Determination of Salbutamol Sulfate in Human Plasma

4.6.1. Optimization Studies

Salbutamol sulphate is a basic compound with pKa = 9.3 and 10.3 (Sutariya et al., 2005). Problems with SS peak shape are fairly common. But there are many simple steps that can dramatically improve the peak shape of problematic SS. These steps are discussed below. Although earlier HPLC methods were accurate and precise for SS determination but the present study is an attempt to develop a HPLC method with better sensitivity.

4.6.1.1. Mobile Phase

During search of an appropriate mobile phase, initially the use of buffer was avoided (Mobile phase 1-5 in Table 3.2). However, to achieve better sensitivity and short analysis time, four different phosphate buffers were employed in the study (Mobile phase 6-13 in Table 3.2). The retention time was found maximum in case of CH_3COONH_4 buffer, followed by NaH_2PO_4, KH_2PO_4 and $(NH_4)H_2PO_4$, respectively while all other HPLC conditions were kept constant. However, following increasing trend was observed on the basis of their peak area as they all produced sharp well resolved peaks; $NaH_2PO_4 < CH_3COONH_4 < KH_2PO_4 < (NH_4)H_2PO_4$. In this attempt, $(NH_4)H_2PO_4$ buffer was selected for further studies as it showed good sensitivity than other three buffers. Instead of CH_3CN as organic solvent, CH_3OH proved itself a good partner of $(NH_4)H_2PO_4$ buffer because it slightly improved sensitivity of the method. Secondly, $(NH_4)H_2PO_4$ concentration used were 47, 57 and 67 mM. Increase in buffer concentration reduced peak tailing for SS and TH and an improvement in peak symmetry was achieved by increasing $(NH_4)H_2PO_4$ concentration from 47 mM to 67 mM. An increase in buffer strength might suppress interactions between SS and stationary phase/silanol groups. Thus, buffer concentration was 67mM at which the resolution and sensitivity of SS and TH was optimum.

Due to high pKa value and low solubility of SS in a medium with high pH, SS has a positive charge on it over the normal useable range of silica based HPLC columns. To prevent ion-exchange interactions between the positively charged SS and negatively charged silanol groups, the mobile phase pH should be low enough to protonate all silanol groups on the silica surface. By this measure, the peak tailing which results from ion-exchange interactions was easily avoided. Therefore, the effect of pH was investigated within the range of 3.0-5.0. No significant change in retention time but slight decrease in sensitivity was observed with an increase in pH. Ultimately, the optimum detection of SS was achieved at pH 3.0 at which resolution factor (Rs) were greater than 2.0 for almost every peak.

Salbutamol sulphate and Triethylamine (TEA), both contain amino group, as shown in Figure 4.36 (A and B), thus TEA (an ion-pairing organic modifier) was added to CH_3OH-$(NH_4)H_2PO_4$ (67mM) as a final step to improve SS peak symmetry. TEA acts as a competing base and minimizes SS-silanol interactions because it pairs with silanol groups of the stationary phase. Thus, quick elution of SS effectively sharpens peaks resulting in improved peak resolution. A 0.5% SDS (displacing agent) was also used as a micellar phase to enhance the solubility of proteins and to minimize binding of SS to plasma proteins. Although it enhanced sensitivity to some extent but variable retention time and slightly broad peaks rejected its use in the finally selected mobile phase.

4.6.1.2. Choice of Internal Standard

The structural formula of tramadol hydrochloride is given in Figure 4.36 (C). It was found the most appropriate internal standard in present analysis because peaks of TH

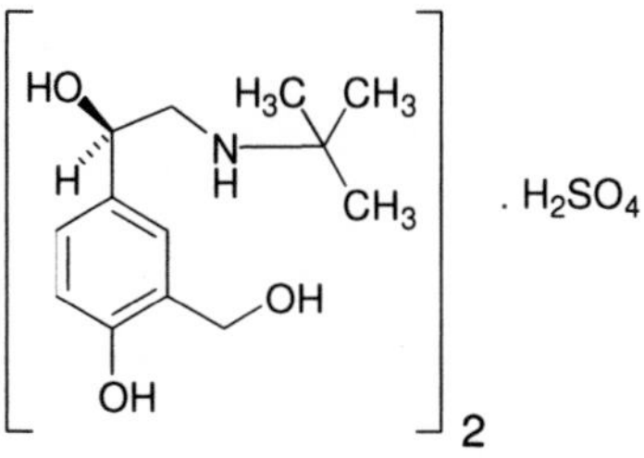

A

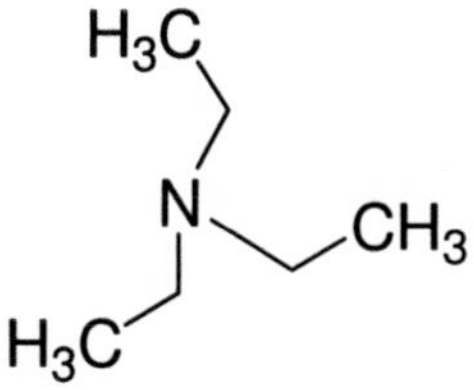

B

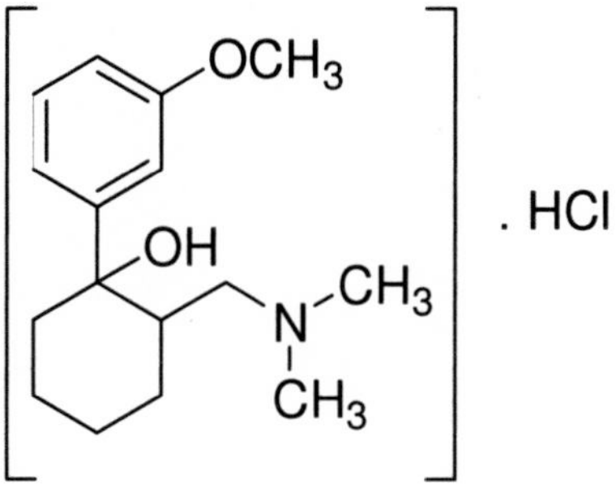

C

Figure 4.36: Structural formulas of salbutamol (A), triethylamine (B) and tramadol (C) and SS had Rs > 2.0 and were symmetrical (asymmetry factor of TH and SS, determined at 10% of total of peak height, were 1.07 and 1.10, respectively). TH eluted without interfering the peaks of plasma and SS as the retention time of SS and TH was 4.1 minutes and 5.2 minutes, respectively. As a result, the run time was set at 15 min/sample. TH also met all the other typical requirements of a compound to be used as an internal standard (e.g. stability, proper solubility).

In the second phase of optimization, different excitation and emission wavelengths were used without varying other parameters. Optimal response was obtained with excitation at 228 nm and emission at 310 nm. Following the above mentioned conditions, a flow rate of 0.7 mL/min showed good resolution of peaks.

As a final phase of optimization strategy, plasma samples were treated with different extracting chemicals i.e. CH_3OH, CH_3CN, DEHP and $HClO_4$. CH_3OH, CH_3CN and $HClO_4$ produced diffused peaks of TH and SS. Where as DEHP showed good resolution (Rs>2.0) of every peak and its nearest ones. DEHP showed better extraction efficiency (75.88-85.52% of SS and 82.28% of TH). 5.5 mL of 0.1M DEHP produced highest extraction efficiency along with 1 mL of 0.5 M HCl for 1.0 mL plasma (Hutchings et al., 1983; Sutariya et al., 2006).

The best conditions for the separation of SS from TH and plasma components are at mobile phase compositions: $CH_3OH:(NH_4)H_2PO_4$ (67mM)(pH 3.0 adjusted with H_3PO_4) : TEA, 50:50:0.02 (v/v/v%) when it was run at a rate of 0.7 mL/min with excitation at 228 nm and emission at 310 nm.

4.6.2. Validation of Method

After the above optimization, a linear calibration curve for SS was obtained in the concentrations range of 0.5-80 ng/mL (n=7). Regression analysis was done on the basis of peak-area of SS (y) in human plasma versus its concentration (x) and a good linearity (0.9989) was observed. The results are presented in Figure 4.37 and Table 4.19. Preparing and analyzing standards of three SS concentrations (low, intermediate and high quality control samples; 0.5, 10, 80 ng/mL) three times, intra- and inter-day relative standard deviation (R.S.D) values were calculated. Intra- and inter-day R.S.D for SS in plasma were less then 4% while Intra- and inter-day accuracy were more than 95% as shown in Table 4.20. These values showed that the proposed method has high repeatability and precision for SS analysis. LOD and LOQ were estimated by signal to noise ratio of 3:1 and 10:1, respectively by following expressions i and ii.

$$LOD = 3.3s / S \qquad \text{(i)}$$

$$LOQ = 10s / S \qquad \text{(ii)}$$

Where "s" is standard deviation of blank readings or standard deviation of regression line and "S" is slope of calibration curve. Based on above equation, the calculated LOD value for SS in plasma was 0.17 ng/mL while LOQ was 0.5 ng/mL as given in Table 4.19. Thus, the present method is also one of the most sensitive ones for SS determination in human plasma (Hutchings et al., 1983; Sagar et al., 1992; Qin et al., 2003). Stability of SS spiked in human plasma was evaluated at the same three concentration levels (0.5, 10, 80 ng/mL) with eleven equally prepared samples at each level. The conditions examined were freeze-thaw cycles, storage in the dark at -20°C for period of 16 days. No significant variation (p>0.05) was observed in peak area even after 16 days than that of the first day.

4.6.3. Pharmacokinetic Studies

The resultant pharmacokinetic (representative mean plasma concentrations versus time) profile of SS in human plasma is shown in Figure 4.38. The corresponding

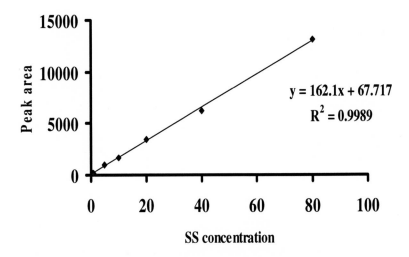

Figure 4.37: Calibration curve (Area of SS peak in spiked plasma versus concentration) of salbutamol sulfate in human plasma

Table 4.19: Regression analysis of calibration line

Serial no.	Parameters	Values of biofluid samples
1	No. of samples	7
2	Concentration range (ng/mL)	0.5-80
3	Regression equation	$y = ax+b$
4	Slope (a)	162.1
5	Intercept (b)	67.717
6	Coefficient of determination (r^2)	0.9989
7	Coefficient of correlation (r)	0.9994
8	LOQ (ng/mL)	0.5
9	LOD (ng/mL)	0.17
10	Extraction efficiency [b] (%)	75.88-85.52

[b] Extraction efficiency = (Peak area of biofluid samples/Peak area of mobile phase samples) × 100

Table 4.20: Summary of intra-day and inter-day Precision and accuracy data (n = 3) for proposed method in human plasma

Serial No.	Added Concentration (ng/mL)	Intra-day			Inter-day		
		Found Concentration [c] (ng/mL)	Precision R.S.D. [d] (%)	Accuracy [e] (bias%)	Found Concentration [c] (ng/mL)	Precision R.S.D. [d] (%)	Accuracy [e] (bias%)
1	0.5	0.5 ± 0.02	3.35	0.56	0.49 ± 0.02	3.86	-1.20
2	1.0	9.86 ± 0.05	0.52	-1.42	9.89 ± 0.09	0.89	-1.10
3	80	80.98 ± 0.43	0.53	1.22	81.06 ± 0.36	0.44	1.31

[c] Found concentration : mean ± standard deviation
[d] Precision R.S.D.(%) : (standard deviation / mean) × 100
[e] Accuracy (bias%) : ((Found concentration − Added concentration) / Added concentration) × 100

pharmacokinetic parameters from noncompartmental analysis of data have been summarized in Table 4.21. The T_{max}, C_{max} and $T_{1/2}$ of SS in the present study were similar, although intake doses were different from those reported in literature (Saleh et al., 2000; Sutariya et al., 2006; Sutariya et al., 2005; Yuan et al., 1998). A typical HPLC chromatogram was obtained and presented in Figure 4.39 which showed SS along with TH in human plasma after 75 minutes of drug administration. Good resolution for every peak was assured by Rs > 1.5.

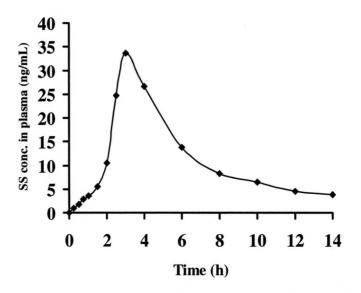

Figure 4.38: Pharmacokinetic profile (n = 24) of salbutamol sulfate in human plasma after single oral administration of a commercially available tablet (8 mg Ventolin SR)

Table 4.21: Pharmacokinetic parameters (n = 24) of salbutamol sulfate in human plasma after single oral administration of a commercially available tablet (8 mg Ventolin SR)

Serial No.	Pharmacokinetic parameters	Observed values
1	Maximum plasma concentration (C_{max})	33.63 ng/mL
2	Time required for maximum plasma concentration (T_{max})	3.0 h
3	Elimination rate constant (K_{el})	$0.14\ h^{-1}$
4	Area under curve (total) ($AUC_{(total)}$)	184.141 ng h / mL
5	Area under first moment curve (total) ($AUMC_{(total)}$)	1476.22 ng h^2 / mL
6	Volume of distribution (V_d)	0.321 mL
7	Plasma half life ($T_{1/2}$)	5.12 h
8	Mean residence time (MRT)	8.02 h
9	Total clearance rate (TCR)	0.0434 l/h

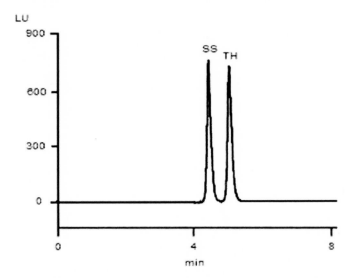

Figure 4.39: A typical chromatograph obtained under the optimized
experimental conditions

4.7. Biowaiver Study of Oral Tabletted Ethylcellulose Microcapsules of a BCS Class I Drug

Entrapment efficiency (%) and production yield (%) of microparticles was found to be approximately 97% and 98%, respectively. The microparticles were whitish, aggregated and irregular in shape (Figure 4.40). Rheological properties of all formulations are expressed in terms of bulk density, taped density, compressibility index, Hausner's ratio and angle of repose (Table 4.2, Page No. 77). It was observed that bulk density decreased with an increase in drug polymer ratio. Present results are in agreement with previous observation where it has been reported that bulk density increased when polymer concentration was decreased (Shariff et al., 2007). Compressibility index of all six formulations is below 15% indicating excellent flow properties. Hausner's ratio and angle of repose were below 1.29 and 30°, respectively, for all formulated microparticles, again indicating their free flow nature (Breghausen et al., 2002).

4.7.1. FTIR spectroscopy

FTIR spectra of SS contained some characteristic and prominent peaks. The spectrum of microparticles also showed amino, hydroxyl and aromatic stretchings at same values as in that of pure SS which confirmed its presence. No significant alteration in the nature of peaks rejected the chances of any strong SS-EC interaction when SS was encapsulated into EC coats. The relevant FTIR spectras are given in Figure 4.5 (Page No. 87).

4.7.2. Thermal Analysis

The specific and well-recognizable thermal profile of drug was observed in a specific temperature range. SS microparticles exhibited same thermal characteristics with reduced sharpness. It revealed a significant reduction of drug crystallinity in the

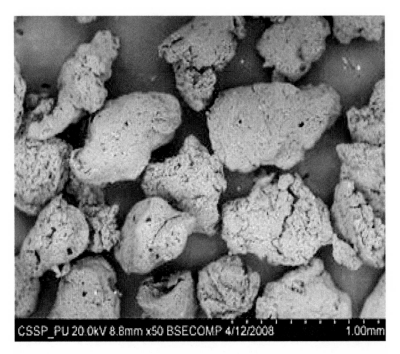

Figure 4.40: Scanning electron micrographs of salbutamol sulpahte-
ethylcellulose microparticles segregated from T_2 formulation
after dissolution

polymer matrix verifying absence of any strong chemical interaction between drug and polymer. Thermal analysis showed good stability of SS in the form of microparticles (Figure 4.6, Page No. 91).

4.7.3. X-ray Diffractometry

X-ray diffractometry revealed amorphous and crystalline nature of pure EC and SS, respectively as shown in diffractograms (Figure 4.7, Page No. 93). However, a decrease in the signal intensity i.e. crystallinity of SS was observed in microparticle form as compared to pure components.

4.7.4. Physical Characterization of Tabletted Microparticles

Physical attributes of tabletted microcapsules were found to be satisfactory. Tablet hardness varied between 8.3 ± 1.2 to 9.5 ± 1.1 kg/cm^2 and friability was less than 0.5% (w/w). The designed tablets showed low weight variation ($< \pm 3.0\%$). The average thickness was 3.87 to 3.89 mm. The results fulfilled the requirements of B.P. (2004).

4.7.5. Mathematical Analysis

4.7.5.1. Model independent approaches

The tabletted microparticles were also evaluated for their release profile in double distilled water, by utilizing different mathematical kinetic models, the difference & similarity factors and one way ANOVA plus Post-Hoc Tests.

Comparison between dissolution profiles of SS tabletted microparticles showed that 60% release of SS was achieved after 4.78, 6.93 and 11.05 hours from T_1, T_2, and T_3, respectively (Figure 4.4, Page No. 86). According to Duncan test, $t_{60\%}$ of all batches of tabletted microparticles lied in the same homogenous group (1:1=1:2=1:3) (p>0.05) whereas Tukey H.S.D. similarized the $t_{60\%}$ of T_1 and T_2 and differentiated them from that of T_3 but not significantly (p>0.05). According to difference factor (f_1) and similarity factor (f_2), the release profiles of following pairs of formulations were different from each other: T_1 versus T_3 and T_2 versus T_3 as their $f_1 > 15.00$ and $f_2 < 50.00$. While T_1 versus T_2 has $f_1 < 15.00$ and $f_2 > 50.00$ that indicates the mutual similarity of compared release profiles but to a very less extent. The results indicated that velocity of drug release was slower from tablets with low polymer concentration i.e. tablet with microparticles having low core to wall ratio and vice versa. It can, therefore, be assumed that decrease in core to wall ratio increased the wall thickness of microparticles and/or decreased the number of surface pores as evident from Figure 4.40. Moreover, it is reported previously that the release of hydrophilic drugs is mainly controlled by permeation through water filled channels within hydrophobic polymer (EC) membrane. It can, therefore, be concluded that both of above mentioned reasons cause a deceleration in diffusion of dissolution medium through these channels that consequently decrease the rate of drug release from tabletted microparticles (Amperiadou and Georgarakis, 1995; Murtaza et al., 2008; Hascicek et al., 2003; Breghausen et al., 2002).

The observed in-vitro drug release profiles from SS tabletted microparticles were biphasic: an initial rapid drug release phase (burst) was followed by slow and prolonged phase. The burst effect may be beneficial because a high initial release produces an instant effect which can be subsequently maintained for a prolonged period by a slower but continuous release of drug. The rank order of tabletted microparticle for percentage drug burst was as: $T_1 > T_2 > T_3$, also visible from Figure 4.4 (Page No. 86). The rapid initial phase of release was thought to occur mainly by dissolution and diffusion of drug entrapped close to or at the surface of microparticles. The second and slower release phase was thought to involve diffusion of drug entrapped within the inner part of polymer matrix by means of aqueous channels of a network of pores. It has been already reported that an initial burst effect in release profile was observed especially when (a) the drug solubility is high, (b) loading dose in the polymeric matrix is large and (c) lack of critical polymer concentration. Additionally, when polymer concentration is low, the hydrated polymeric matrix would be highly porous leading to rapid diffusion of drug from polymeric matrix (Erden and Celebi, 1996; Singh and Robinson, 1990).

4.7.5.2. Model dependent approaches

In order to get meaningful information, the whole drug release profiles were evaluated kinetically and the best fit of release profiles to zero order, first order, Higuchi, Hixson-Crowell and Korsmeyer-Peppas models was investigated. Model with highest co-efficient of determination (R^2) was judged to be a more appropriate model for dissolution data. The release profiles from all formulations were best explained by Higuchi model due to highest linearity, followed by zero order and first order, respectively. It suggests that drug release is controlled by diffusion of drug through pores and not through swollen EC. From Korsmeyer-Peppas model, it is found that the mode of release from all tabletted microparticles was anomalous (non-Fickian, a combination of diffusion and erosion mechanism) diffusion. The application of release profiles to Hixson-Crowell equation indicated a change in surface area and diameter of formulation with progressive dissolution of matrix as a function of time.

4.7.6. Estimation of Swelling and Erosion of Tabletted Microparticles

The optimum formulation after putting into dissolution apparatus undergoes swelling and erosion continuously with time (h) as clear from Figure 4.8 (Page No. 94). This phenomenon is responsible for gradual release of drug from tabletted microcapsule matrix. It also confirms anomalous diffusion of SS from tabletted microparticles.

4.7.7. Bioavailability Studies

The corresponding pharmacokinetic parameters from non-compartmental analysis of the data of all four formulations have been summarized in Table 4.22. Application of ANOVA ascertained insignificant ($p > 0.05$) difference in the values of C_{max} and T_{max} of M_1, M_2, M_3 and reference formulations. However, $AUC_{(total)}$ and $AUMC_{(total)}$ of T_3 is significantly ($p < 0.05$) different from M_1, M_2 and reference formulations which may be due to the fact that T_3 is most sustained formulation than other three and stays for longer time in circulatory system and thus results in higher $AUC_{(total)}$ and $AUMC_{(total)}$ of T_3.

4.7.8. In vitro - In vivo Correlation for Tabletted Microparticles

A good correlation between the dissolution and pharmacokinetic data was observed. IVIVC was determined by drawing plots between drug absorbed (%) and drug dissolved (%) at same time points for all three formulations. A high value of determination coefficient ($R^2 = 0.9224$, 0.945, 0.9363 and 0.9694 for T_1, T_2, T_3 and reference formulations, respectively) suggested good correlation between in vitro and in vivo profiles (Figure 4.41). This correlation shows that dissolution profile can be utilized as a predictive tool for in vivo data. Figure 4.42 shows a faster SS dissolution rate than its absorption rate. It elaborates that gastric emptying is a rate controlling factor in the absorption of SS from tabletted microcapsules (Ferrari et al., 1993).

4.7.9. Validation of Method

The prediction error was found to be less than 9.68% which is within the limits.

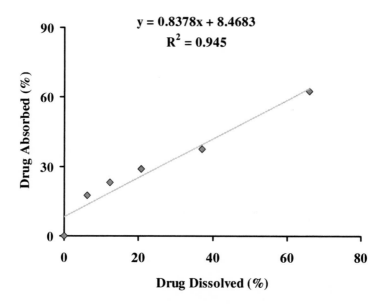

$$y = 0.8378x + 8.4683$$
$$R^2 = 0.945$$

Figure 4.41: A rectangular coordinate plot between drug absorbed (%) and drug dissolved (%) for an optimum formulation (T_2) of salbutamol sulphate-ethylcellulose tabletted microcapsules

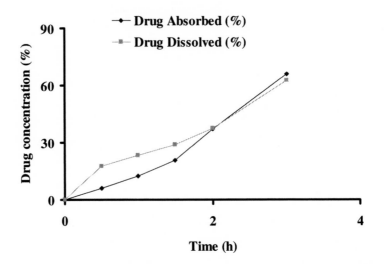

Figure 4.42: A rectangular coordinate plot of cumulative drug absorbed (%) and drug dissolved (%) versus time (h) for an optimum formulation (T_2) of salbutamol sulphate-ethylcellulose tabletted microcapsules

Table 4.22: Pharmacokinetic parameters of salbutamol sulphate after a single sustained release oral dose of different formulations of salbutamol sulphate administered to human volunteers (N = 24)

Serial No.	Pharmacokinetic parameters	Observed values For T_1	Observed values For T_2	Observed values For T_3	Reference
1	Maximum plasma concentration (C_{max}, ng/ml)	36.06	33.63	28.43	35.74
2	Time required for maximum plasma concentration (T_{max}, h)	3.0	3.0	3.0	3.0
3	Area under curve (total) ($AUC_{(total)}$, (ng h / ml)	210.70	208.75	238.71	215.69
4	Area under first moment curve (total) ($AUMC_{(total)}$, (ng h^2 / ml)	1502.05	1593.79	2260.95	1506.20
5	Percent prediction error	< 10.00	< 10.00	< 10.00	< 10.00

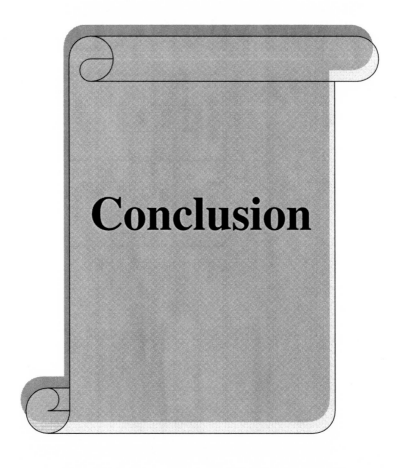

Conclusion

5.1. Salbutamol Sulphate-Ethylcellulose Microparticles: Formulation and In-Vitro Evaluation with Emphasis on Mathematical Approaches

This study has explored that the non-solvent addition coacervation technique is an appropriate method to microencapsulate salbutamol sulpahte into ethylcellulose coats. It could be concluded that the variation observed in entrapment efficiency, production yield, mean particle size and drug release behavior among formulations are the result of drug polymer ratio employed. No strong chemical interaction between drug and polymer was found. These results may suggest the potential application of ethylcellulose microparticles as a suitable sustained release drug delivery system. Therefore, it is possible to formulate a single-unit, sustained-release oral dosage form of salbutamol sulpahte at least twice in every 24 hours using ethylcellulose.

5.2. Microencapsulation of Tramadol hydrochloride and Physicochemical Evaluation of Formulations

Non-solvent addition coacervation technique is an appropriate method to prepare tramadol hydrochloride-ethylcellulose microparticles and the variation observed in entrapment efficiency, production yield, mean particle size and the drug release behavior among formulations are the result of drug polymer ratio employed. This study may suggest the potential application of ethylcellulose microparticles as a suitable multi-unit sustained release drug delivery system after every 12 hours.

5.3. Preparation and Physicochemical Characterization of Diclofenac sodium Microparticles

Non-solvent addition phase separation was found to be a successful technique for the microencapsulation of diclofenac sodium with ethylcellulose. The characterization of drug, polymer and microparticles explained that it is a physical method for the microencapsulation of drug as no chemical interaction was found between drug and polymer. Diclofenac sodium is a model sparingly hydrophilic drug that paves the way to encapsulate other sparingly hydrophilic drugs into ethylcellulose for development of their sustained release dosage forms.

5.4. Mathematical Comparative Characterization of Microencapsulated Diclofenac sodium, Salbutamol sulphate and Tramadol hydrochloride

This study has assessed that the non-solvent addition coacervation technique is an appropriate method to microencapsulate drugs with different solubilities (TH, SS and DS) into the EC coats. It could be concluded that the variation observed in entrapment efficiency, production yield, mean particle size and drug release behavior among formulations are the result of nature of drugs (i.e. water solubility or insolubility) and the drug polymer ratio employed. The results may also suggest the potential application of ethylcellulose microparticles as a suitable sustained release drug delivery system as it does not affect the nature of drugs and no chemical bonding establishes between drug and polymer during this method. Therefore, it is possible to formulate a single-unit, sustained-release dosage form of TH, SS and DS for oral administration at least once every 12 hours using this polymer (i.e. EC).

5.5. A Comparative Study of Various Microencapsulation Techniques: Effect of Polymer Viscosity on Microcapsule Characteristics

In conclusion, there is no significant difference in terms of the physical properties of microcapsules prepared by these three techniques. However, this study explains that CTC is an appropriate method to microencapsulate salbutamol sulpahte into ethylcellulose shells because of its good entrapment efficiency, sustained drug release behavior, rapidness and ease. It could be concluded that variation observed in entrapment efficiency, production yield, mean particle size and drug release behavior among formulations are the result of drug polymer ratio employed. These results may suggest the potential application of ethylcellulose microparticles as a suitable sustained release drug delivery system. Therefore, it is possible to formulate a single-unit, sustained-release oral dosage form of salbutamol sulpahte at least twice in every 24 hours using ethylcellulose.

5.6 Optimization and Validation of a New and Sensitive Reverse Phase HPLC Method with Fluorescent Detection for the Determination of Salbutamol Sulfate in Human Plasma

In the present study, a new sensitive and specific RP-HPLC method has been developed, optimized and validated for SS estimation in human plasma using FLD and isocratic elution. Optimization elaborated that the mobile phase composition and excitation and emission wave lengths of FLD are as crucial parameters as flow rate for reproducible and quantitative determination of SS. The method was found to be linear over an analytical range of 0.5-80 ng/mL with LOD = 0.17 ng/mL and LOQ = 0.5 ng/mL, respectively. An excellent accuracy (>95%) and precision (<4%) was achieved. In conclusion, this method can be used successfully in routine drug monitoring and pharmacokinetic studies.

5.7 Biowaiver Study of Oral Tabletted Ethylcellulose Microcapsules of A BCS Class I Drug

Non-solvent addition coacervation technique is a good method to encapsulate salbutamol sulpahte into the ethylcellulose shells. Moreover, oral tabletted ethylcellulose microcapsules are good sustained release drug delivery system for biowaiver study of BCS class I drugs. Present results also certify that the encapsulated salbutamol sulphate (with 1:1 and 1:2 drug-polymer ratios) used in this study is bioequivalent to commercial salbutamol sulphate and moreover, encapsulation did not interfere with the efficacy of salbutamol sulphate. However, smart scrutiny of plasma drug concentration-time profiles in healthy human volunteers exhibited that encapsulation produces a delay in absorption of salbutamol sulphate.

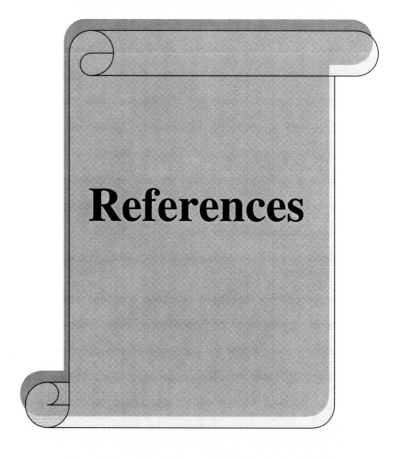

References

REFERENCES

1. Acosta N., Aranaz I., Peniche C. and Heras A. (2003). Tramadol Release from a Delivery System Based on Alginate-Chitosan Microcapsules. Macromol. Biosci. 3: 546–551.

2. Al Frayh A., Abba A., Iskandarani A., Shaker D. S., Zai-Toun F., Shahrabani L., Khan M., Riachy M. and Dham R. (2008). Establishing Therapeutic Bioequivalence of a Generic Salbutamol (Butalin®) Metered Dose Inhaler to Ventolin®. Biomed. Res. 19: 61-68.

3. Al-Taani B. M. and Tashtoush B. M. (2003). Effect of Microenvironment pH of Swellable and Erodable Buffered Matrices on the Release Characteristics of Diclofenac Sodium. AAPS Pharmscitech. 4: E43-E49.

4. Altman R. A., Hochberg M. C., Moskowitz R. W. and Schnitzer T. J. (2000). Recommendations for the Medical Management of Osteoarthritis of the Hip and Knee, 2000 Update. Arthritis Rheum. 43: 1905-1915.

5. Amperiadou A. and Georgarakis M. (1995). Controlled Release Salbutamol Sulphate Microcapsules Prepared By Emulsion Solvent-Evaporation Technique and Study on the Release Affected Parameters. Int. J. Pharm. 115: 1-8.

6. Bakan J. A. (1986). Microencapsulation. Lachman L., Lieberman H. A., Kanig J. I., The Theory and Practice of Industrial Pharmacy. 2nd Ed. Philadelphia: Lea & Febiger. P. 412-429.

7. Banakar U. V., Hanson W. A., Lathia C. D., Paul A. M., Vitticaden S. J., Wood J. H., (1992). Pharmaceutical Dissolution Testing, Marcel Dekker, Inc., New York, USA.

8. Banker G. S. and Anderson N. R. (1987). Tablets. Lachman L., Lieberman H. A., Kanig J. I., The Theory and Practice of Industrial Pharmacy. 2nd Ed. Philadelphia: Lea & Febiger. P. 416-419.

9. Barik B. B., Ray S., Goswami N., Gupta B. K. and Ghosh L. K. (2001). Preparation and in Vitro Dissolution of Isoniazid from Ethylcellulose Microcapsules. J. Acta Polo. Pharm-Drug Res. 58: 65-68.

10. Barret S.B., (2004). Bioavailability and Bioequivalence Studies. in Pharmacokinetics in Drug Development: Clinical Study Design and Analysis. Ed. Bonate P and Howard D. American Association of Pharmaceutical Scientist. USA.

11. Benita S., (2006). Microencapsulation – Methods and Industrial Applications, 5th Edition, Taylor & Francis, New York, USA.

12. Bhanja R. S. and Pal T. K. (1989). In-Vitro Diffusion Kinetics of Salbutamol Sulphate from Microcapsules Coated with Eudragit RS 100. Boll. Chim. Farm. 128: 281-283.

13. Biju S. S., Saisivam S., Maria N. S., Rajan G. and Mishra P. R. (2004). Dual Coated Erodible Microcapsules for Modified Release of Diclofenac Sodium. Eur. J. Pharm. Biopharm. 58: 61–67.

14. Boulton D. W. and Fawcett J. P. (1996). Enantioselective Disposition of Salbutamol in Man Following Oral and Intravenous Administration. Br. J. Clin. Pharmacol. 41: 35-40.

15. BP. (2004). Appendix XII G. Uniformity of Weight (Mass). London: British Pharmacopoeia Commission. P 1.

16. Breghausen S. W., Schote U., Frey M. and Schmidt F. (2002). Comparison of Microencapsulation Techniques for the Water Soluble Drugs Nitenpyram and Clomipramine HCl. J. Control. Release. 85: 35-43.

17. Cutler D.J. (1978). Linear System Analysis in Pharmacokinetics. Pharmacokinet. Biopharm. 6: 265-282.

18. Davis S.S. (2005). Formulation Strategies for Absorption Windows. Drug Discov. Today. 10: 249-257.

19. Davis S.S., Hardy J.G. and Fara J.W. (1986). Transit of Pharmaceutical Dosage Forms through the Small Intestine. Gut 27: 886-892.

20. Dillard R.L., Eastman H. and Fordtran J.S. (1965). Volume-Flow Relationship during the Transport of Fluid through the Human Small Intestine. Gastroenterology 49: 58-66.

21. Dokoumetzidis A. and Macheras P. (2006). A Century of Dissolution Research: from Noyes and Whitney to the Biopharmaceutics Classification System. Int. J. Pharm. 321: 1-11.

22. Dressman J.B., Amidon G.L., Reppas C. and Shah V.P. (1998). Dissolution Testing as a Prognostic Tool for Oral Drug Absorption: Immediate Release Dosage Forms. Pharm. Res. 15: 11-22.

23. Dressman J.B., Berardi R.R., Dermentzoglou L.C., Russel T.L., Schmaltz S.P., Barnet J.L. and Jarvenpaa K. (1990). Upper Gastrointestinal pH in Young Healthy Men and Women. Pharm. Res. 7: 756-761.

24. Dressman J.B., Butler J., Hempenstall J. and Reppas C. (2001). The BCS: Where Do We Go from Here? Pharm. Techol. July: 68-76.

25. Dressman J.B., Vertzoni M, Goumas K. and Reppas C. (2007). Estimating Drug Solubility in the Gastrointestinal Tract. Adv. Drug Del. Rev. 59: 591-602.

26. El-Gindy A., Emara S. and Shaaban H. (2007). Development and Validation of Chemometrics-Assisted Spectrophotometeric and Liquid Chromatographic Methods for the Simultaneous Determination of Two Multicomponent Mixtures Containing Bronchodilator Drugs. J. Pharm. Biomed. Anal. 2007. 43: 973-982.

27. Emami J. (2006). in Vitro - in Vivo Correlation: From Theory To Applications. J. Pharm. Pharm. Sci. 9: 169-189.

28. Erden N. and Celebi N. (1996). Factors Influencing Release of Salbutamol Sulphate from Poly (Lactide-Co-Glycolide) Microspheres Prepared By Water-In-Oil-Water Emulsion Technique. Int. J. Pharm. 137: 57-66.

29. Erram S. V., Fanska C. B. and Asif M. (2006). Determination of Albuterol Sulfate and its Related Substances in Albuterol Sulfate Inhalation Solution, 0.5% by RP-HPLC. J. Pharm. Biomed. Anal. 40: 864-874.

30. Fagerholm U. (2007). Evaluation and Suggested Improvements of the Biopharmaceutics Classification System. J. Pharm. Pharmacol. 59: 751-757.

31. FDA (2000). Guidance For The Industry: Analytical Method Validation, US Food and Drug Administration, Center For Drug Evaluation and Research (CDER), Rockville, MD.

32. FDA Guidance for Industry, (1995). Immediate-Release Solid Oral Dosage Forms, Scale-Up and Postapproval Changes: Chemistry, Manufacturing, and Controls, in Vitro Dissolution Testing, and In Vivo Bioequivalency Documentation. U.S. Department of Health and Human Services Food and Drug Administration Center for Drug Evaluation and Research (CDER).

33. FDA Guidance for Industry, (1997). Extended Release Oral Dosage Forms: Development, Evaluation, and Application of in Vitro/in Vivo Correlations. Ed. Rockville, MD: Food and Drug Administration U.S. Department of Health and Human Services Food and Drug Administration Center for Drug Evaluation and Research (CDER).

34. FDA Guidance for Industry, (2000). Waiver of in Vivo Bioavailability and Bioequivalence Studies for Immediate-Release Solid Oral Dosage Forms Based on a Biopharmaceutics Classification System. Ed. Rockville, MD: Food and Drug Administration. U.S. Department of Health and Human Services Food and Drug Administration Center for Drug Evaluation and Research (CDER).

35. Forsdahl, G. and Gmeiner, G. (2004). Quantification and Stability of Salbutamol in Human Urine. J. Sep. Sci. 27:110-114.

36. Fowler P. D., Shadforth M. F., Crook P. R. and John V. A. (1983). Plasma and Synovial Fluid Concentrations of Diclofenac Sodium and its Major

Hydroxylated Metabolites during Long Term Treatment of Rheumatoid Arthritis. Eur. J. Clin. Pharmacol. 25: 389-394.

37. Goodman L. S., Gilman A., Brunto L. L., Lazo J. S., Parker K. L., (2006). Goodman & Gilman's, The Pharmacological Basis of Therapeutics. 11th Edition, McGraw Hill Publishers, USA.

38. Grass G. M. and Sinko P. J. (2002). Physiologically-Based Pharmacokinetic Simulation Modelling. Advanced Drug Delivery Reviews. 54: 433-451.

39. Gray V., Dressman J.B., (1996). Simulated Intestinal Fluids, TS-Change to pH 6.8. Pharmacopoeial Forum. 22: 1943-1945.

40. Grond S. and Sablotzki A. (2004). Clinical Pharmacology of Tramadol. Clin. Pharmacokin. 43: 879-923.

41. Halabi A., Ferrayoli C., Palacio M., Dabbene V. and Palacios S. (2004). Validation of A Chiral HPLC Assay for (R)-Salbutamol Sulfate. J. Pharm. Biomed. Anal. 34: 45-51.

42. Hascicek C., Gonul N. and Erk N. (2003). Mucoadhesive Microspheres Containing Gentamicin Sulphate For Nasal Administration: Preparation and in Vitro Characterization. II Farmaco. 58: 11-16.

43. Higuchi T. (1963). Mechanism of Sustained Action Medication. Theoretical Analysis of Rate of Release of Solid Drugs Dispersed in Solid Matrices. J. Pharm. Sci. 52: 1145-1149.

44. Hindle M., Peers E. M., Parry-Billings M. and Chrystyn H. (2003). Relative Bioavailability of Salbutamol to the Lung Following Inhalation via a Novel Dry Powder Inhaler and A Standard Metered Dose Inhaler. Br. J. Clin. Pharmacol. 43: 336 – 338.

45. Hixson A. W. and Crowell J. H. (1931). Dependence of Reaction Velocity upon Surface and Agitation: I-Theoretical Consideration. Ind. Eng. Chem. 23: 923-931.

46. Hongfei L., Tianhui S., Feiqian Y., Xin Z., Hong G. and Weisan P. (2007). The Investigation of The Pharmacokinetics of Pulsatile-Release Salbutamol Sulfate with Ph-Sensitive Ion Exchange Resin as the Carriers in Beagle Does. Chem. Pharm. Bull. 55: 480-481.

47. Isabel D., Moises K., (2004). Flow-Injection Spectrophotometeric Determination of Salbutamol with 4-Aminoantipyrine. Talanta. 64: 1233-1236.

48. Jianli Z., Youxuan X., Xin D. and Moutian W. (2006). Quantitation of Salbutamol in Human Urine by Liquid Chromatography–Electrospray Ionization Mass Spectrometry. J. Chromatogr. B. 831: 328–332.

49. Jin O. B., Jing L. D., Willy R. G. B. and Joris R. (2005). A Simple Method for the Study of Salbutamol Pharmacokinetics by Ion Chromatography with Direct Conductivity Detection. Talanta. 65: 1–6.

50. Khatun M., Islam S. M. A., Akter P., Quadir M. A. and Reza M. S. (2004). Controlled Release of Naproxen Sodium from Eudragit RS100 Transdermal Film. Dhaka Uni. J. Pharm. Sci. 3: 1-10.

51. Koester L. K., Ortega G. G., Mayorga P. and Bassani V. L. (2004). Mathematical Evaluation of In-Vitro Release Profiles of Hydroxypropylmethylcellulose Matrix Tablets Containing Carbamazepine Associated To B-Cyclodextrin. Eur. J. Pharm. Biopharm. 58: 177-179.

52. Korsmeyer R. W., Gurny R., Doelker E., Buri P. and Peppas N. A. (1983). Mechanisms of Solute Release from Porous Hydrophilic Polymers. Int. J. Pharm. 15: 25-35.

53. Kortejarvi H. (2008). Modelling and Simulation Approaches for Waiving in Vivo Pharmacokinetic Formulation Studies. Academic Dissertation.

54. Kuksal A., Tiwary A. K., Jain N. K. and Jain S. (2006). Formulation and in Vitro, in Vivo Evaluation of Extended- Release Matrix Tablet of Zidovudine: Influence of Combination of Hydrophilic and Hydrophobic Matrix Formers. AAPS Pharmscitech. 7: E1-E9.

55. Kumbar S. G., Kulkarni A. R. and Aminabhavi T. M. (2002). Crosslinked Chitosan Microspheres for Encapsulation of Diclofenac Sodium: Effect of Crosslinking Agent. J. Microencapsul. 19: 173-180.

56. Lee C. R., Mctavish D. and Sorkin E. M. (1993). Tramadol, a Preliminary Review of its Pharmacodynamic and Pharmacokinetic Properties and Therapeutic Potential in Acute and Chronic Pain States. Drugs. 46: 313-340.

57. Lennernas H. and Abrahamsson B. (2005). The Use of Biopharmaceutic Classification of Drugs in Drug Discovery and Development: Current Status and Future Extensions. J. Pharm. Pharmacol. 57: 273-285.

58. Loden H., Pettersson C., Arvidsson T. and Amini A. (2008). Quantitative Determination of Salbutamol in Tablets by Multiple-Injection Capillary Zone Electrophoresis. J Chromatogr A. [In Press]

59. Loo J. C. K. and Riegelman S. (1968). New Method for Calculating the Intrinsic Absorption Rate of Drugs. J. Pharm. Sci. 57: 918-928.

60. Martindale-The Extra Pharmacopoeia (2002). 33rd Ed., Sean C Sweetman; P. 770-773.

61. Morgan D. J., Paull J. D., Richmond B. H., Wilson-Evered E. and Ziccone S. P. (1986). Pharmacokinetics of Intravenous and Oral Salbutamol and its Sulphate Conjugate. Br. J. Clin. Pharmacol. 22: 587–593.

62. Murthy T. E. J. K. and Chowdary K. P. R. (2005). Formulation and Evaluation of Ethyl Cellulose-Coated Diclofenac Sodium Microcapsules: Influence of Solvents. Ind. J. Pharm. Sci. 67: 216-219.

63. Najafabadi A. R., Vatanara A. R., Gilani K. and Tehrani M. R. (2005). Formation of Salbutamol Sulphate Microparticles Using Solution Enhanced Dispersion By Supercritical Carbon Dioxide. Daru. 13: 1-5.

64. Nefedova Y., Nagaraj S., Rosenbauer A., Muro-Cacho C., Sebti S. M. and Gabrilovichs D. I. (2005). Regulation of Dendritic Cell Differentiation and Antitumor Immune Response in Cancer by Pharmacologic-Selective Inhibition of the Janus-Activated Kinase 2/Signal Transducers and Activators of Transcription 3 Pathway. Cancer Res. 65: 9525-9535.

65. Ohannesian L., Streeter A. J., (2002). Handbook of Pharamaceutical Analysis, Volume 11, Marcel Dekker, Inc., New York, USA.

66. Pachuau L., Sarkar S. and Mazumder B. (2008). Formulation and Evaluation of Matrix Microspheres for Simultaneous Delivery of Salbutamol Sulphate and Theophylline. Trop. J. Pharm. Res. 7: 995-1002.

67. Physician Desk Reference, (2001). Thomson Reuters, Times Square, New York, USA.

68. Polli J. E. and Rekhi G. S. (1996). Methods to Compare Dissolution Profiles. Drug Inform. J. 30: 1113-1120.

69. Qin, Y., Zou, Y., Liang, M., Yu, Q., Huang, Y., Li, T. and Xu, X. (2003). Determination of Salbutamol in Human Plasma by Column Switching HPLC with UV Detection. Sichuan Da Xue Xue Bao Yi Xue Ban. 34:576-579.

70. Ritschel W. A., Kearns G. L., (2004). Handbook of Basic Pharmacokinetics ---- including clinical applications. 6th Edition, American Pharmaceutical Association, USA.

71. Ritter J. M., Lewis L. D. and Mant T. G. K. (1999). A Text Book of Clinical Pharmacology. 4th Edition. Awan Publishers, India.

72. Rosa B., Jordi S., Rosa V., Kenneth D. F., Alan R. M., Magí F., Marta M. and Xavier D. L. T. (2000). Discrimination of Prohibited Oral Use of Salbutamol from Authorized Inhaled Asthma Treatment. Clin. Chem. 46: 1365-1375.

73. Rowe R. C., Sheskey R. J. and Weller P. J. (2003). Handbook of Pharmaceutical Excepient. 4th Edition. 237-241.

74. Rowland M. and Tozer T. N. (1995). Clinical Pharmacokinetics. Concepts and Applications, 3rd Edition. Williams & Wilkins, Waverly Company, USA.

75. SA B., Bandyopadhyay A. K. and Gupta B. K. (1996). Effect of Microcapsule Size and Polyisobutylene Concentration on the Release of Theophylline from Ethylcellulose Microcapsules. J. Microencapsul. 13:207-218.

76. Sah H. (1997). Microencapsulation Techniques Using Ethyl Acetate As Disperse Solvent: Effects of its Extraction Rate on the Characteristics of PLGA Microspheres. J. Control. Release. 47:233-245.

77. Sajeev C., Vinay G., Archna R. and Saha R. N. (2002). Oral Controlled Release Formulation of Diclofenac Sodium by Microencapsulation with Ethylcellulose. J. Microencapsul. 19: 753-760.

78. Saleh, M. L., Koh, Y. M., Tan, S. C. and Aishah, A. L. (2000). Clean Up, Detection and Determination of Salbutamol in Human Urine and Serum. Analyst. 125:1569-1572.

79. Salman M. A., Salin A., Onur M. A., Oge K., Kassab A. and Aypar U. (2003). Tramadol Encapsulated into Polyhydroxybutyrate Microspheres: in Vitro Release and Epidural Analgesic Effect in Rats. Acta Anaesthesiol. Scand. 47: 1006-1012.

80. Schiller C., Frohlich C. P., Giesmann T., Siegmund T., Monnikes H., Hosten N. and Weitschies W. (2005). Intestinal Fluid Volumes and Transit of Dosage Forms As Assessed By Magnetic Resonance Imaging. Aliment. Pharmacol. Ther. 22: 971-979.

81. Shariff A., Manna P. K., Paranjothy K. L. K. and Manjula M. (2007). Entrapment of Andrographolide in Cross Linked Alginate Pellets: H. Physicochemical Characterization to Study the Pelletization of Andrographolide. Pak. J. Pharm. Sci. 20: 1-9.

82. Sherri L. M., Priya S. and Charles S. W. (2007). Stereoisomer Analysis of Wastewater Derived-Blockers, Selective Serotonin Re-Uptake Inhibitors, and Salbutamol by High-Performance Liquid Chromatography–Tandem Mass Spectrometry. J. Chromatogr. A. 1170: 23–33.

83. Sheu M. T., Chou H. L., Kao C. C., Liu C. H. and Sokoloski T. D. (1992). Dissolution of Diclofenac Sodium from Matrix Tablets, Int. J. Pharm. 85: 57–63.

84. Singh J. and Robinson D. H. (1990). Controlled Release Captopril Microcapsules: Effect of Ethylcellulose Viscosity Grade on The in Vitro Dissolution from Microcapsules and Tabletted Microcapsules. J. Microencapsul. 7: 67-76.

85. Sirichai S. and Khanatharana P. (2008). Rapid Analysis of Clenbuterol, Salbutamol, Procaterol, and Fenoterol in Pharmaceuticals and Human Urine by Capillary Electrophoresis. Talanta. 76: 1194-8.

86. Soppimath K. S., Kulkarni A. R. and Aminabhavi T. M. (2001). Encapsulation of Antihypertensive Drugs in Cellulose-Based Matrix Microspheres: Characterization and Release Kinetics of Microspheres and Tabletted Microspheres. J. Microencapsul. 18: 397-409.

87. Sutariya V. B., Mashru R. C., Sankalia M. G. Y. and Sankalia J. M. (2006). Liquid Chromatographic Determination and Pharmacokinetics Study of Salbutamol Sulphate in Rabbit Plasma. Ars Pharm. 47: 185-197.

88. Taha E. I., Zaghloul A. A., Samy A. M., AL-Saidan S., Kassem A. A. and Khan M. A. (2004). Bioavailability Assessment of Salbutamol Sulfate Suppositories in Human Volunteers. Int. J. Pharm. 279: 3-7.

89. Thombre A.G. (2005). Assessment of the Feasibility of Oral Controlled-Release in an Exploratory Development Setting. Drug Discov. Today. 17: 1159-1166.

90. Ungell A. L., Nylander S., Bergstrand S., Sjoberg Å. and Lennernas H. (1998). Membrane Transport of Drugs in Different Regions of the Intestinal Tract of The Rat. J. Pharm. Sci. 87: 360-366.

91. United State Pharmacopoeia 27 – National 22 (USP-NF), (2004). Webcom Limited, Toronto, Canada.

92. Valenzuela B., Lopez-Pintor E., Perez-Ruixo J. J., Nacher A., Martın-Villodre A. and Casabo V. G. (2006). Modelling Intestinal Absorption of Salbutamol Sulphate in Rats. Int. J. Pharm. 314: 21–30.

93. Veng-Pedersen P. and Modi N. B. (1992). An Algorithm for Constrained Deconvolution Based Reparameterization. Pharm. Sci. 81: 175-180.

94. Wagner J.G. and Nelson E. (1964). Kinetic Analysis of Blood Levels and Urinary Excretion in the Absorptive Phase after Single Doses of Drug. J. Pharm. Sci. 53: 1392-1403.

95. Wilson C.G. and Washington N. (1989). The Stomach: Its Role in Oral Drug Delivery. In Physiological Pharmaceutical: Biological Barriers To Drug Absorption. Edited Rubinstein MH. Chichester, UK, Ellis Horwood: 47-70.

96. World Health Organization (WHO) (2006). Multisource (Generic) Pharmaceutical Products: Guidelines on Registration Requirements to Establish Interchangeability. Annex7. WHO Technical Report Series, No. 937.

97. Yamuda T., Ohnishi H. and Machida Y. (2001). Sustained Release Ketoprofen Microparticles with Ethylcellulose and Carboxymethylethylcellulose. J. Control. Release. 75: 271-282.

98. Yazan Y., Demirel M. and Guler E. (1995). Preparation and in Vitro Dissolution of Salbutamol Sulphate Microcapsules and Tabletted Microcapsules. J. Microencapsul. 12: 601-607.

99. Yu L.X., Crison J.R. and Amidon G.L. (1996). Compartmental Transit and Dispersion Model Analysis of Small Intestinal Transit Flow in Humans. Int. J. Pharm. 140: 111-118.

100. Zhang Z. Y., Ping Q. N. and Xiao B. (2000). Microencapsulation and Characterization of Tramadol-Resin Complexes. J. Control. Release. 66: 107-133.

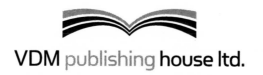
 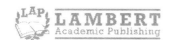 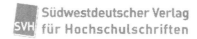

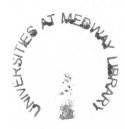

Lightning Source UK Ltd.
Milton Keynes UK
171298UK00001B/107/P

9 783838 384122